More Praise for Acres of SKIN

"...A well-researched, convincing study...effectively blends the prisoner's own lurid stories with a researcher's dispassionate overview."

—*Publishers Weekly*

"...A devastating picture of U.S. medical experimentation and the men, educational institutions, and drug companies that carried it out."

—*Booklist*

"...A thorough account of questionable medical experimentation...shocking.... Essential for students of medical ethics."

—*Library Journal*

"...An ugly tale of outrageous abuse of prisoners at Philadelphia's infamous Holmsburg prison.... A seminal work."

—Linn Washington, Jr., *The Philadelphia Tribune*

"*Acres of Skin* is a powerful and impassioned exposé of the dark side of American medicine. Most damning is Hornblum's documentation of the callous indifference of prison authorities, politicians, the U.S. Military, and the so-called watchdogs of the medical profession to the hideous and dangerous experiments performed by physicians who violated their sacred oath to heal, not harm, their patients. A most important book."

—Sheldon Harris, author of *Factories of Death: Japanese Biological Warfare, 1932-1945 and the American Cover-Up* (Routledge)

"...Painful to read, but it must be read—not only for its historical significance but also for what it can still teach us about the conduct of medical research in the contemporary world. For Allen

Hornblum's compelling account of what transpired within Holmsburg prison is, sadly, only a chapter in an ongoing story."

—Jay Katz, Professor of Law, Medicine and Psychiatry, Yale Law School

"Allen Hornblum's *Acres of Skin* does for Holmsburg what David Rothman's *Willowbrook Wars* did for Willowbrook and James H. Jones' *Bad Blood* did for Tuskegee. Each show how the authority of science has been used to effect officially sanctioned exploitation of the vulnerable. Part of the tragedy is that we must wait decades for its public exposure."

—John Kleinig, Director of the Institute for Criminal Justice Ethics at the John Jay College of Criminal Justice

Acres of
SKIN

Human Experiments at
Holmesburg Prison

A True Story of Abuse and Exploitation in the
Name of Medical Science

Allen M. Hornblum

Routledge
New York   London

Published in 1998 by

Routledge
29 West 35th Street
New York, NY 10001

Published in Great Britain by
Routledge
11 New Fetter Lane
London EC4P 4EE

Text Design by Debora Hilu

Library of Congress Cataloging-in-Publication Data
Hornblum, Allen M.
    Acres of skin : human experiments at Holmesburg Prison : a
true story of abuse and exploitation in the name of medical science
/ Allen M. Hornblum.
      p. cm.
    Includes bibliographical references and index.
    ISBN 0-415-92336-0 (pbk. : alk. paper)
    1. Holmesburg Prison. 2. Human experimentation in
medicine—Pennsylvania—Philadelphia. 3. Prisoners—
Medical care—Pennsylvania—Philadelphia. 4. Convict
labor—Pennsylvania—Philadelphia. 5. Dermatology—
Research—Pennsylvania—Philadelphia. I. Title.
[R853.H8H67 1998b]
174' .28—dc21
                                  98-43691
                                  CIP

To My Mother

I sit on a man's back, choking him and making him carry me. And yet assure myself and others, that I am very sorry for him and wish to lighten his burden by all possible means. Except, by getting off his back.

—Leo Tolstoy

Contents

Part Four
The End of Experimentation at Holmesburg

The Nuremberg Code

1. The voluntary consent of the human subject is absolutely essential. This means that the person involved should have legal capacity to give consent; should be so situated as to be able to exercise free power of choice, without the intervention of any element of force, fraud, deceit, duress, overreaching, or other ulterior form of constraint or coercion; and should have sufficient knowledge and comprehension of the elements of the subject matter involved as to enable him to make an understanding and enlightened decision. This latter element requires that before the acceptance of an affirmative decision by the experimental subject there should be made known to him the nature, duration, and purpose of the experiment; the method and means by which it is to be conducted; all inconveniences and hazards reasonably to be expected; and the effects upon his health or person which may possibly come from his participation in the experiment. The duty and responsibility for ascertaining the quality of the consent rests upon each individual who initiates, directs or engages in the experiment. It is a personal duty and responsibility which may not be delegated to another with impunity.

2. The experiment should be such as to yield fruitful results for the good of society, unprocurable by other methods or means of study, and not random and unnecessary in nature.

3. The experiment should be so designed and based on the results of animal experimentation and a knowledge of the natural history of the disease or other problem under study that the anticipated results will justify the performance of the experiment.

4. The experiment should be so conducted as to avoid all unnecessary physical and mental suffering and injury.

5. No experiment should be conducted where there is an a priori reason to believe that death or disabling injury will occur; except, perhaps, in those experiments where the experimental physicians also serve as subjects.

6. The degree of risk to be taken should never exceed that determined by the humanitarian importance of the problem to be solved by the experiment.

7. Proper preparations should be made and adequate facilities provided to protect the experimental subject against even remote possibilities of injury, disability, or death.

8. The experiment should be conducted only by scientifically qualified persons. The highest degree of skill and care should be required through all stages of the experiment of those who conduct or engage in the experiment.

9. During the course of the experiment the human subject should be at liberty to bring the experiment to an end if he has reached the physical or mental state where continuation of the experiment seems to him to be impossible.

10. During the course of the experiment the scientist in charge must be prepared to terminate the experiment at any stage, if he has probable cause to believe, in the exercise of the good faith, superior skill, and careful judgement required of him, that a continuation of the experiment is likely to result in injury, disability, or death to the experimental subject.

Introduction

On a sweltering September morning in 1971, I took my first appre-
hensive steps inside the Philadelphia Detention Center to teach an
adult literacy class. The prison bustled with activity; no one
seemed to be locked up. Prisoners—most of them black, dressed in
light blue cotton shirts over dark navy pants—moved in a dozen
different directions, without apparent guidance or supervision. A
few of the inmates displayed the same fear my eyes must have
shown, but most swaggered brazenly, cursing and joking as if the
steel and cinderblock facility that held them captive were just
another neighborhood hangout. To a white, middle-class, 23-year-
old who had just completed graduate school on Philadelphia's
lush and conservative Main Line, the detention center was as
remote as the far side of the moon.

As I toured the institution, I gradually adjusted to the foul odors,
the jeers and hooting from prisoners, the suspicious glares from
guards, and to a supercharged intercom that alternated commands
and announcements with Top-40 R&B tunes. The most peculiar
sight that first day, the sight to which I could not and never did
adjust, is the subject of this book. Scores of men, bare chested in the
oppressive heat, were covered with gauze pads and adhesive tape.
As they ambled between the cell blocks, gymnasium, and dining
hall, I wondered about the violence that had caused the multiple
wounds covering their backs, shoulders, and arms. Were they knife
wounds from a prison brawl? Was the prison so unsafe? I looked
more closely and gradually noticed that the gauze and tape were
laid out in an oddly symmetrical pattern. A few days later, I asked
a guard on A Block, John Reeves, about my discovery. He answered
matter-of-factly: "They're part of the perfume test being run by the

University of Pennsylvania."[1] I struggled to reconcile the incongruity of unshaven, tattoo-covered criminals testing delicate and expensive feminine fragrances, and shot a doubtful look at the guard. But he assured me it was true. The "perfume experiments"— and numerous other experiments that neither he nor anyone else seemed to understand (including the test subjects)—had been going on for a long time; in fact, they had begun many years before he had started working as a correctional officer in the early 1960s.

My dismay surprised Reeves, to whom the research program had become an accepted part of the prison culture. "Look," he said, "you and I wouldn't do it, sell ourselves for chump change to some strange college doctors, but inmates are crazy. And this is their only way to make money in jail."[2]

I remained puzzled by the experiments as well as by my own reaction to them. Why did research experiments on the inmates trouble me? Why didn't they trouble the guards or the inmates themselves? I asked many inmates: Why did they participate in such risky ventures? Did the tests frighten them? Did the tests leave any lasting scars or cause any lasting problems? The answers were uniformly the same: Yes, they were concerned about the experiments—some were quite frightened of them—but they were desperate for money and this was the way to earn it.

I got to know one of the inmates, "Wash," who recruited students for my adult literacy course. When I questioned him about volunteering for the medical tests, he said, "Mr. Hornblum, these patch tests ain't gonna hurt me. Besides a little itching, it don't hurt none. I know which of these tests are safe. And anyway, I done put everything through these veins you can shoot through a needle. Why'm I gonna worry 'bout some patches when I got years of smack in me? Besides, I need the money. This place gets pretty stale without some spendin' money for commissary."[3]

In time, I learned that even more research experiments were underway at the House of Correction, just across Pennypack Creek from the detention center, and still more at Holmesburg Prison, where a sophisticated dermatology lab had been established, and three-quarters of the inmate population were said to be involved in the testing program. Both prisoners and guards could recite a list of experiments Holmesburg hosted, tests involving toothpaste, deodorant, shampoo, skin creams, detergents, liquid diets, eye drops, foot powders, and hair dye, all seemingly benign but accompanied by constant biopsies and frequently painful procedures. Occasionally, someone would whisper that LSD and cancer experiments were taking place as well.[4] Because the inmate volunteers seemed satisfied with the monetary incentives, and the guards and social workers were unconcerned, I muffled my concern and focused on recruiting new candidates for high school diplomas.

Unbeknownst to both prisoners and staff, a wave of moral, legal, and public opposition to the ethics of performing experiments on institutional volunteers was about to envelop the scientists and doctors who orchestrated these experiments. In just a few short years, both the style and substance of medical research would change. As one scholar of this "controversial transformation" described it, the image of the physician as sole judge of appropriate patient care was yielding to the image of "an examining room so crowded that the physician had difficulty squeezing in and [a] patient [was] surrounded by strangers."[5] By the mid-1970s, the vast majority of medical experiments on institutionalized populations was over. Thereafter, doctors who wanted to accomplish similar experimental results on humans "had to jump through 100 hoops of varying government regulations."[6]

But questions remain: Why did such a process flourish in postwar America and apparently not in other industrialized nations? Why did human experiments on vulnerable, institutionalized populations go on so long in the United States? And why were so many public officials and watchdog groups unmoved when Nazi experiments on captive populations had made such exploitation so repugnant?

In 1947, seven distinguished German doctors and scientists were sentenced to death and nine others were committed to long prison terms by the International Military Tribunal on war crimes at Nuremberg, Germany. These men had performed medical experiments on concentration camp inmates that, by any standards, were horrendous. The Nuremberg Code, crafted by American jurists after the "Doctors' Trial" in August 1947, established ten principles, including the rights and autonomy of experimental subjects and the corresponding responsibility of physicians to ensure informed consent. Intended "to satisfy moral, ethical and legal concepts in the conduct of research,"[7] the Code strove to safeguard the health and rights of individuals who chose freely to participate in human research.

The Nazi doctors who were brought to trial offered a vigorous defense based on revelations that, from the early part of this century, American physicians had conducted similar nontherapeutic experiments on prisoners. These uncomfortable disclosures neither exonerated the German doctors nor caused the American medical community to re-examine its policies. In fact, the opposite occurred. Rather than embracing the Nuremberg Code, the American medical establishment considered it a "good code for barbarians, but an unnecessary code for ordinary physician-scientists" like themselves.[8] Over the next two decades, the number of American medical research programs that relied on prisoners as subjects rapidly expanded as zealous doctors and researchers, grant-seeking universities, and a burgeoning pharmaceutical industry raced for greater market share. Society's marginal people were, as they had always been, the grist for the medical-pharmaceutical mill, and prison inmates in particular would become the raw materials for postwar profit-making and academic advancement. As Senator Edward Kennedy said soberly during senate hearings on the subject in 1973, "Those who have borne the principal brunt of research—whether it is drugs or even experimental surgery—have been the more disadvantaged people within our society; have been the institutionalized, the poor, and minority members."[9]

Recent revelations about city, state, and federal governments' complicity in such experiments clearly expose the weakness of America's past bioethical standards. Experiments were approved for state and county facilities, drug tests were approved by the FDA, and military-intelligence agencies initiated their own tests.

We harrangued and executed Nazi doctors for experiments that forced humans to drink seawater, to be placed in icewater, to be castrated, to be infected with spotted fever and other pathogens, and to undergo painful limb transplant experiments,[10] but at the same time we found it justifiable to inject hospital patients with plutonium without their consent,[11] and to observe hundreds of poor, black sharecroppers in Macon County, Alabama, as they withered away from syphilis while withholding effective treatment.[12] The use of human materials to expand medical knowledge in nonlethal experiments at Auschwitz, Dachau, and Ravensbruck was not significantly different from giving retarded orphans breakfast cereal in milk laced with radioactive calcium at the Walter E. Fernald State School in Massachusetts.[13]

Domestically, the well-being of research subjects was viewed as important, but, in the eyes of medical practitioners, not as important as scientific advancement. Many in the medical community believed the vigorous protection of research subjects, combined with the Hippocratic ideal of *primum non nocere* ("first of all, to do no harm") was too restrictive a code of professional ethics, especially for physicians who had not committed the pseudo-scientific outrages of the concentration camps. The result was a marginalization of the Code and the creation of an ethical loophole that allowed physicians to pursue a pragmatic and utilitarian course while de-emphasizing the Code's critical provisions of informed consent by autonomous subjects. Since research was seen to have social importance, doctors could easily avoid the Nuremberg Code's prescriptive safeguards and aggressively pursue their individual goals.

Though the physicians following this course may have escaped public disclosure and embarrassment at the time, history may be less forgiving. The historical investigation of human-subjects research in America is a relatively recent development, but scholars have already taken sides over the issue of individual culpability:[14] How critical can contemporary scholars be of actors and actions that occurred many decades ago? How significant are such issues as "conflicting obligations," "factual ignorance," and "culturally induced moral ignorance," in hobbling judgments of wrongdoing and blameworthiness?[15] And if wrongdoing is established, does blameworthiness necessarily follow? These questions inform and impel the writing of this book.

More than a century ago, Claude Bernard, the famous French physician and founder of modern experimental medicine, declared:

> The principle of medical and surgical morality, therefore, consists in never performing on man an experiment which might be harmful to him to any extent, even though the result may be highly advantageous to science, that is, to the health of others.[16]

By the early twentieth century, however, Bernard's high-minded principle was being honored more in the breach than in the observance, a fundamental canon to which one paid lip service. Instilled with a sense of omniscience, but lacking a moral compass, the best and brightest in America's medical community put scientific interest and benefit to future patients above the health of their subject-patients. By the mid-twentieth century, doctors were injecting prisoners with polio, tuberculosis, and cancer cells; performing various burn and radiation studies; subjecting volunteers to an assortment of powerful hallucinogenic and psychotropic drugs; and smearing everything from powerful solvents and acids to dioxin on compliant, unwitting convicts. For some among the medical elite, people in prisons had become a means to an end. Maurice H. Pappworth, a British physician and early critic of unethical research, must have felt very lonely indeed when, in 1967, he called for the medical profession to rectify some of its worst abuses:

> No physician is justified in placing science or the public welfare first and his obligation to the individual, who is his patient or subject, second. No doctor, however great his capacity or original his ideas, has the right to choose martyrs for science or for the general good.[17]

The stories of some institutionalized populations subjected to research experiments have appeared in ethical journals and various texts, but the disturbing tales of the prisoners who suffered the experimental research have been largely untold, devalued experiences of people of low social status. The 1963 case of the Jewish Chronic Disease Hospital, in which Dr. Chester Southam deliberately injected two dozen senile hospital patients with a live cancer virus in order to study the role the body's immune system plays in defense against cancer, has become infamous; Southam's similar experiments (albeit with a degree of informed consent) eight years earlier on eight times as many subjects at Ohio State Penitentiary are relatively unknown. Likewise, while the Fernald and Willowbrook experiments—in which retarded children were purposefully exposed to radioactive isotopes and hepatitis, respectively—have become much-studied landmarks of the postwar period, comparable events at Holmesburg Prison and dozens of penal institutions have been forgotten.

Acres of Skin is an attempt to rectify that omission, to show how American prisoners were exploited in the name of medical science just as senile hospital patients, retarded orphans, and other institutionalized populations were exploited in postwar America. This story will finally give voice to a segment of society that "volunteered" their minds and bodies so that physicians could acquire scientific advancement, fame, and fortune; volunteers who were forgotten and tossed aside—in a utilitarian age in which ambition and profit became the ultimate good, and the pursuit of scientific knowledge took precedence over the rights of individual human beings.

The story centers on Holmesburg Prison—the largest of Philadelphia's county jails—which became the epicenter of troubling research. Doctors and medical students who trained there went on to successful careers and reproduced the Holmesburg model in other prisons in other states. The inmates themselves remained so much medical waste, still incarcerated and less whole than before.

Holmesburg was for many years the professional base for the career of the story's central character, Dr. Albert M. Kligman, architect of the prison's experimental research program. Considered at once a genius, a medical pioneer, and the archetypal entrepreneur,

Kligman is credited with both "unilaterally [raising] dermatology to its high status today"[18] and changing dermatology from a sub-specialty of medicine to a cosmetic industry by "[pandering] to the worst instincts in medicine."[19] Certainly, Holmesburg Prison was a paradise for an ambitious research dermatologist. Looking back in 1966, Kligman recalled his awe when he first visited the prison: "All I saw before me were acres of skin. It was like a farmer seeing a fertile field for the first time."[20] Kligman wasted no time cultivating and harvesting his acres. Widely quoted in newspapers and magazines, discoverer of the fabulously successful skin cream, Retin-A®, Kligman, by sheer force of will—and what many call his innate brilliance for making money from medicine—created a glittering career that vaulted his name far beyond the walls of Holmesburg.

Not so his human guinea pigs who sacrificed their health and comfort to experimental medicine. They remained behind, to nurse mutely their scars and unpleasant memories. The scars and memories linger. But these men are no longer mute.

A Note on Sources

Though the origin of this book goes back over a quarter of a century to my first startled impressions of the Holmesburg medical experiments, research for this book did not begin until 1993. Initial interviews with former inmate test subjects increased my interest in the subject, but their lack of knowledge as to just what chemicals and substances they were exposed to or the purposes of the experiments meant that a thorough historical investigation would be required.[1] Compounding the problem at this earliest stage of my research was the lack of cooperation from key elements—the physicians and medical technicians—who knew some of the answers to the Holmesburg riddle. Their responses to my inquires ran the gamut from fear and indignation, to a need to contact their attorneys. Curiously, the better-informed were the most reluctant to talk about the Holmesburg experiments. Though I would continue to explore personal leads, and in fact, interviewed hundreds of prisoners, doctors, and others who had come in contact with the Holmesburg experiments, it was obvious that acquiring objective documentation of the prison research would be essential if the true story was ever to be revealed.

The Urban Archives of Temple University proved a crucial resource for old newspaper accounts and photographs of Holmesburg Prison during this stage of the investigation. Though the articles from that period and after further illuminated the depth and scope of the experiments, it was still surface material that raised more questions than it answered.

It was at this point that I decided to orchestrate a thorough search of government documentation on the Holmesburg medical research program. The Freedom of Information Act proved an invaluable resource in attaining these important and highly informative documents. F.O. I. A. submissions resulted in acquiring thousands of pages of material that revealed the little known, but more questionable experiments on prisoners. Because of the wide-ranging nature of the studies undertaken at the prison, the F.O.I.A. process necessitated sending requests to numerous governmental departments. Department of Defense documents concerning the U.S. Army's chemical warfare studies; the Central Intelligence Agency's role in similar studies; the Nuclear Regulatory Commission's files on radioactive isotope use; the Environmental Protection Agency's files on the dioxin experiments; and the Food and Drug Administration's files on the DMSO investigation, among other issues all contributed to gaining a more nuanced and complete understanding as to what took place at Holmesburg Prison.[2] It can be said without exaggeration that without the Freedom of Information Act, this book would never have been possible.

Needless to say, however, other individuals and resources contributed mightily to this project. Dr. Susan Lederer, a scholar who has written extensively on the subject of human experimentation in America supplied me with critical material concerning the use of prisoners as test subjects prior to World War II. Dr. James Ketchum, a psychiatrist who devoted many years to the Army's Chemical Corps, was gracious enough to partake of numerous interviews and offer me copies of his personal files on the Army's Holmesburg experiments. Anne Diestel, archives specialist, at the Federal Bureau of Prisons supplied me with valuable information concerning federal prisoner participation in medical research. And Suzanne White Junod and Carolann Hooton proved exceedingly helpful in extracting hard-to-gain files from the Food and Drug Administration. Alan Lawson offered me his copies of the U.S. Senate's 1973 Hearings on Human Experimentation. Assistant U.S. Attorney Ken Jost supplied me with hundreds of pages of legal material concerning the federal government's investigation of Ortho Pharmaceutical. And Philadelphia attorney Lawrence Cohan allowed me to explore his files on one of the few lawsuits filed against the experimenters.

In addition, the medical libraries of the University of Pennsylvania, Hahnemann University, and the College of Physicians were perused extensively for relevant journal articles that originated as clinical studies at Holmesburg Prison. Old medical periodicals proved to be a gold mine of interesting and revealing information regarding the practice of research medicine a generation ago. More revelations concerning the darker side of human experimentation in America will no doubt surface in future years as scholars begin a more thorough investigation of this partially explored field of study.

Part One

THE SUBJECTS, THE DOCTORS,

AND THE

EXPERIMENTS

One

"The Money Was Good and the Money Was Easy."

They marched six of us, three blacks and three whites, all the same age, late twenties–early thirties, into this one room of the trailer. They told us to strip down and put on these white, cotton pullovers with three-quarter sleeves and elastic bands around the waist. Some of us were getting pretty nervous now, especially when we saw the syringes on the table.

I never did drugs, it wasn't my thing. I was into chasing women and crime, but no drugs. Good-looking women and nice cars, that's how I got my high.

The attendants all looked professional in white smocks and stethoscopes. They lined us up and gave us our shots. I learned later that the shot I got was based on my height and weight. One of the doctors told us to go into the rec room and relax. I went in and sat down on some plastic furniture. There was heavy padding under the shag rug on the floor. I felt fine. I picked up a pack of playing cards that was on the table and asked another guy, "Do you want to play some gin rummy?" He said, "Okay," and as I dealt the cards I could feel it coming on. The room started to spin around. I looked at my hand, and it looked like there were 30 or 40 cards there.

It was only three to five minutes after the shot, but I was on a real trip. I started to see double and triple, and the room was really spinning pretty good. I went back to when I was four or five years old and playing with little kids. Then I was about seven years old and going to school and I was in a classroom with all the other little children I used to know. All the old faces came back to me. Then I went from 7 to 14 or 15 and my first serious girlfriend. We were going to dances, making out in the back seat of the car. It took me right up until my twenties. It was a good trip.[1]

I

The year was 1964, the location was Holmesburg Prison in Philadelphia, and inmate Al Zabala had just become a test subject for the U.S. Army in one of its tests of chemical agents. Serving a one-year sentence for burglary, the 27-year-old Zabala had originally expressed fear at being part of an experiment, but he gradually overcame his misgivings—for a fee. His personal story is typical of the thousands of American prisoners who decided to sell themselves as experimental subjects during the postwar expansion of medical research. This chapter offers an opportunity for those who contributed their bodies to science, but never achieved fame or fortune, to tell their side of the story: To explain why they chose to be, and what it was like to be, a Holmesburg guinea pig.

Born in South Philadelphia, Al Zabala was raised in New Jersey with his two sisters and three brothers. His parents separated in the mid-1950s, and his mother remarried twice while scratching out a living operating a series of small restaurants. In June 1954, he joined the Navy and got his first taste of life behind bars. While stationed in Pensacola, Florida, Zabala served three months in the brig for theft. For the next ten years he was able to stay clear of prison, but he was far from being a law-abiding citizen. Zabala and his friends stole cars and sold them to chop shops, each car bringing between $500 and $600. After a few years, they stepped up to burglary, starting with smash-and-grabs at fur stores on the Main Line, Philadelphia's affluent western suburb.

"There were three of us," he recalls, "a wheelman and two to swing the baseball bats. Smash the store window and grab seven or eight furs before anybody knew what happened. Then we got into jewelry stores. Same deal. Before they put those heavy steel grates on the windows, it was easy."[2]

In 1963, Zabala was imprisoned again, this time in Philadelphia. Jobs in jail were rare, competition for them was tough, and the pay was poor. "My first jail job was as a goon in OBS [the Psychological Observation Unit]. I put straightjackets on the patients in Holmesburg's psych unit. I soon heard about the U of P [University of Pennsylvania] studies and the good pay they offered. They had all kinds of tests—foot powder tests, eye drop tests, face creams, underarm deodorant, toothpaste, liquid diets, and more. It was easy money. You could make $10 to $300 a test depending on how long it lasted."

Despite the pay, Zabala was still wary of the university's experiments and decided instead to take an assistant technician job with the unit. "A friend of mine worked for them and he recommended me. They gave me a test to see if I could read and write. There was a reading comprehension test, an interview, and then I was hired." Zabala was taken to H Block, the cell block where all the tests were administered. There were "freezers, refrigerators, and all kinds of food, real street food. We got a lot of special treatment."

As an inmate worker for the University of Pennsylvania, Zabala received about $40–$50 a month and the opportunity to be part of any test he wanted. For six months, Zabala watched and decided what to do. "Lots of crazy stuff went on in there." Everything made him suspicious; samples were labeled by "numbers and codes" and if he asked what a specific cream or lotion was, or who was testing it, the technicians replied "We don't know" or "We can't tell you."

"Lots of men were burned or scarred and wanted to sue, but they had signed releases and waivers and thought they couldn't," Zabala says. He, too, came away with a prominent scar, a permanent reminder of his days as a "chemist" in the U of P research unit. His account of that incident is interesting for the light it sheds on the wide latitude given to inmate workers in the clinical research program.

> We were given jars marked A, B, C, D...with percentages of 2%, 8%, 4%....We had to mix the creams together and then put them on the inmates. This one time, I got the job to mix the chemicals for the test and I wasn't paying attention to what I was doing. But I still had the sense to test it on myself [before I used it] and it burned a hole the size of a thumbnail in [the skin of] my right forearm. It hurt like hell. If I [had] put that stuff on an inmate, he would have come back at me with a pipe or a shank.

Despite potential dangers, Zabala could not remain immune to the lures of the testing program. "It was something to do, the best game in town. The money was good and the money was easy." He first tried a deodorant test. He chose the one he thought had the least chance of harming him, and says it was funny watching other prisoners smell his armpits and look for signs of irritation. He was a bit uneasy that the underarm lotion was unlabeled, but the $25 he received each week smothered his concern. He went on to test hand and body lotions and soon realized the program's full financial potential. "Three or four tests at a time could mean real easy money. Foot powder tests and deodorants would bring you $100 per month, and hand creams a buck a day. You could be making $300 to $400 a month." Though meager by outside-world standards, these wages were incredible by ordinary pay scales in prisons of the 1960s. Workers received 15 cents a day to make shoes, knit socks and shirts, sew trousers, and work in the plumbing shop.[3] For Zabala, who had had a decent paying job with the psych unit, the appeal of big money was enough to tempt and convert an opponent of human experimentation.

"I was scared of other tests," recalls Zabala, "medications and eyedrops [with] no labels on them. They looked nasty." Zabala put aside his reluctance to try anything other than topical ointments when he heard talk around the prison that a special study for the Army was starting and that the pay would dwarf anything the subjects had seen so far. A volunteer could make somewhere between $1,000 and $1,500. Zabala decided to check it out.

He was given "a 15-minute interview [in which] white-coat professionals from the University of Pennsylvania asked questions about his age, place of birth, family history of mental illness, or health problems." A couple of weeks later he was asked to fill out a three-page questionnaire and was surprised to receive $25. That was followed by a second interview with a psychologist and a psychiatrist, and an additional $50. Zabala felt he was making out pretty well and he hadn't done anything yet. "They were sucking [me] in with all the money," he says.

Shortly thereafter, Zabala's group of six inmates along with three other similarly sized groups were given thorough physical examinations, more exacting than any they had ever received. The day before the actual test, they were given a "talk" that described a test of "experimental stuff," but nothing too specific. The test subjects were asked to sign a paper, a kind of "release" from any damage claims. In return, they were given $300. "The money closed the deal."

Al Zabala believes he was given an injection of a substance "ten times stronger than LSD" and remained in the trailer for seven days. Except for the "trip" he has no recollection of his actions during that period. His room was completely padded, walls and floors, and two corners of the ceiling held video and audio equipment. "The microphone was about the size of a pack of cigarettes and the surveillance camera half the size of a shoe box." A "peep slot" in the door allowed the testing staff to observe the subjects at any time. Toward the end of his stay, the medical staff peppered him with questions: Who are you? Where are you? What are you doing here? Zabala says, "I figured what they gave us was pretty damn potent. I got the impression that [one of the technicians who kept an eye on me] didn't like the study, didn't approve of it."

> I wasn't right for a month after the test. I was real subdued and quiet. I had problems swallowing food and a constantly dry throat. They put me on a liquid diet until I could swallow whole food again. When we finally came back to population, all the guys on the study had to wear badges that said we were not responsible for our actions and if we acted up to get U of P personnel to come and get us. We had to wear these badges for a month and once a week talked to the psychs. They made us take paperwork and association tests to measure our psychological condition.

Some prisoners, according to Zabala, had such bad reactions to the drugs that staff had to restrain them and give them antidotes.

> [A few] guys came back to population and didn't remember their names. Guys would fade in and out of consciousness....Some guys beat themselves up and punched themselves in the head. Some of the guys told me they had violent, ugly trips—dogs as big as horses, worms like alligators—horrible trips, being eaten by giant spiders, living in the 13th century. One guy said he was hung and killed.

For a few years Al Zabala's body would periodically break out in "strawberry rashes," but overall, he felt fine, helped by the fact that he walked out of Holmesburg "$1,500 richer because of the drug study." Nearly a decade later, however, he began to have second thoughts. Two incidents concerned him and gave rise to troubling questions about the Army study. The first occurred in 1973, when Zabala locked himself in the bedroom of his sister's house for three days and refused to come out. He did not eat, sleep, or wash during that period and did not respond to his sister's pleas to unlock the door. When he finally came out he had no recollection of the prior three days. His sister encouraged him to see a doctor, but he refused. He claims never to have had such an incident again, but he may have. According to William Robb, a convicted murderer serving a life term at the State Correctional Institution at Pittsburgh, he saw Zabala experience something similar in the mid-1970s.[4] Robb had escaped from a series of prisons, and before leaving the area, he decided to share a farewell drink with Zabala at a neighborhood bar. As soon as they sat down, Zabala started to behave in an odd manner and fainted. Robb thought Zabala might have a brain tumor, but Zabala passed it off as a weird aftereffect of the tests at Holmesburg. He never took these incidents seriously until the late 1970s, when newspaper "articles began to appear, describing the extent of the Holmesburg medical studies." Then he began to wonder if the tests had "changed the molecules in [his] body or affected [his] chromosomes."

II

William Robb also has a clear recollection of the Holmesburg experiments and describes the different varieties of tests in the following letter:

> In 1970 [and] 1971, I participated in three different types of tests....Two of the[m], nicknamed "The Patch Tests" by inmates, dealt with...the experimentation of new products not yet released to the general public....The first Patch Test...was one [that] tested lotions, creams, skin moisturizers, and suntan products. The procedure for these tests [was] as follows: A grid, made from thick strips of white hospital tape was fixed to the

upper portion of an inmate's back shoulders. The grid consisted of about 20 squares. In each one of these squares a dab of lotion was applied and the inmate's back was exposed to different temperatures from a sunlamp. The exposure to the sunlamp lasted anywhere from 15 to 30 minutes, after which each square was inspected for degree of blistering or other adverse reactions....The grid was then covered with a large solid piece of tape (to prevent tampering by the inmate) and the inmate was returned to his cell. This test lasted about 30 days and once a day...the inmate was called back over to the lab and exposed to the sunlamp. After about five days of the sunlamp, there [were] sections of the...skin that were burnt a deep brown and the skin started to peel, itch, and blister. If a certain square became too damaged it was covered over with a permanent piece of tape and the tests continued on the grid.[5]

According to numerous interviews, the patch test was one of the most common tests performed on the inmates. The resulting patchwork quilt design left on the prisoner's backs and shoulders remained for years after they had left Holmesburg. "My back is all marked up [with] bad blackheads and scars," complains Withers Ponton a 79-year-old lifer convicted of homicide in the late 1960s.[6] An example of someone who repeatedly signed on as a human guinea pig, he went through "over 50 tests" during his "40 months" in the county jail and figures he "made a couple grand" during that period. Ponton took part in "at least 25 biopsy tests" and says he has "about 6 different spots and 24 different marks" on his back that "are still there after 25 years." He says he got "a needle in the shoulder each week and then a biopsy where they would take a portion out." He received "$5 for each test site and $30 for all." Ponton's ability to endure the pain and suffering from a wide range of tests is remarkable, considering his reaction to his first experiment. "That first test nearly killed me it was so painful. I nearly went through the wall. I had a patch put on my back that covered a large area. It was a 10-day test and I wasn't allowed to take a shower," he says. He received $10 or $15.

One of the more unusual experiments that Withers Ponton agreed to was what he calls the "gauze test." With no anesthetic, he lay on a table while "two young doctors from the University of Pennsylvania" cut two 1-inch incisions on each side of his lower back. They inserted gauze pads into the wounds, and then stitched up the incisions. Ten days later, Ponton returned, the doctors reopened one wound, removed the gauze pad, and restitched the wound. After another 10 days, Ponton was brought back for the same procedure on the other incision. He was never told the purpose of the exercise and accepted $20 for his trouble—"$10 for each cut." He's still angry that "now I got these scars all over my back."

"I looked like a checkerboard with patches and skin discoloration on my arms, back and chest," says Ron Keenan, a lifer at Graterford Prison, who spent 34 months at Holmesburg in the late 1960s while awaiting trial for the murder of a policeman.[7] "I was on a lot of suntan tests because I was light-skinned," but the patch tests "really irritated my back....I [had] burn blisters for months." "I was afraid of the patch test, it was like a tattoo," says Billy Allison, a Graterford inmate.[8] "One year later I got on one [study] and I was sorry I did."

Both inmates and guards say you can recognize a Holmesburg inmate decades later by the distinctive scars from skin burns and patch tests. "If you ever saw the guys on the beach," says Captain James Kinslow, who started working in Holmesburg in 1965, "you would know where the hell they've been."[9] Joseph Dade, a retired Philadelphia deputy sheriff and former Holmesburg guard, says, "Guys sold themselves for a few bucks. Guys looked like zebras when the patches came off."[10] Correctional officer Hank Brame uses a different metaphor. For many, the patches became "a symbol of status or achievement, much like stripes on the sleeve of a soldier. Some of those patches took the skin clear off," but the inmates thought their willingness to subject themselves to such experiments added to their macho status in jail.[11]

One academic study that examined why prisoners volunteered as subjects for medical research experiments did indeed find that "nearly all the non-volunteers believed that volunteering for such an enterprise was an 'act of courage.'"[12] With the passage of time, however, the idea of bravery has receded in the minds of many former Holmesburg inmates interviewed. In fact, not one of the inmates—either those who volunteered or those who refused—mention the extra respect accorded the test subjects.

Though many test subjects are now embarrassed by their distinctive, discolored skin, aesthetics were clearly subordinate to the need for money at the time of the tests. Payment for skin tests varied according to the substance and the sponsoring pharmaceutical company; the test William Robb describes paid approximately $35. "A king's ransom," Robb argues, "for an inmate trying to raise bail money."[13]

Robb took part in a second patch test that the prisoners ultimately referred to as "The Douche Patch Test," because he says "an inmate-nurse who worked in the lab discovered that the lotion being tested was a new product [to be] marketed for female hygienic vaginal use." This test was similar to the others, but in this case the grid was placed on the forearm and there was no sunlamp. According to Robb, results could be felt "within hours after having the solution placed within the small squares." His skin was examined each day, and after 30 days he was paid $60.

As Robb remembers the third test,

> [it] seemed to be the favorite among inmates...[and] became known as "The Milkshake Test." Each day selected inmates went to H Block and drank "a rich, creamy-tasting 'milkshake,'" something like today's diet drinks. The test lasted anywhere from 30 to 90 days depending on the results [from] each...inmate. Two types of milkshakes were given out to the inmates: a vanilla-flavored concoction for the thinnies and a chocolate-flavored one for the fatties....At first, [there was] a problem with the milkshake test: the first three weeks, the fatties gained weight and the thinnies lost weight and suffered dehydration. There was a mix-up...where the milkshakes were being passed out....It took a while for the lab to work out the bugs.

Robb had no ill effects from the milkshake test and attempted to do an extra 60 days. Not only was he well paid—inmates were paid "$100 for a 60-day and $150 for a 90-day test"[14]—but the liquid diet also allowed him to stay out of "the dreaded mess hall," site of inmate fights and several bloody skirmishes between prisoners and guards.

Not all inmates liked the liquid-diet drink. "It made me sick," says Ron Keenan.[15] "Boy, that stuff was horrible." He drank the milkshakes for ten weeks and earned $200, but claims most inmates found the drink distasteful and "cheated" by purchasing "swag [contraband] sandwiches" from friends who worked in the mess hall. Even for those prisoners who enjoyed the taste, the milkshake drinks were generally not enough to sustain men for an entire day, and it is probable that many inmate-volunteers compromised the tests.

Whether the University of Pennsylvania doctors and test administrators were aware of it, cheating was common among the test subjects and prisoners were resourceful in avoiding test constraints. Hoping to avoid discomfort and irritation, they took off the taped grid as soon as they returned to their cells from H Block. Guards said it was not unusual to go into an inmate's cell and find long strips of adhesive tape hanging from the wall. Thomas Sims, 18 years old when he first entered Holmesburg in 1966, confirms that "some guys took [the grid] off and hung it on the wall....Those doctors were running a game on us, so we ran a game on them."[16] Tom McGevren, a former lifer who entered Holmesburg in 1972, concurs: "To some degree it was a joke because we wore the patches on the testing block [but] took them off and hung them up when we got back to our cell."[17] McGevren participated in three patch test studies and was paid $25 for each. He saw some inmates get "really messed up" in the tests, like the time "some guys on a shampoo test started to lose their hair." Still, he was just concerned about one thing: "the money."

Between the patch and diet tests, many experiments were compromised by wily inmates. Curiously, no one—including the prisoners, the medical administrators, or the pharmaceutical companies sponsoring the tests—seemed to care. "Inmates ran a con game on them," says Al Bronstein, a long-time prison reform advocate and former Director of the National Prison Project. "Some of these studies were scientifically worthless."[18]

III

Other tests generated results opposite to their design. A prime example was the experiment Branham referred to: a "new dandruff treatment" that was tested during the summer of 1967. At the time, Dr. Sigmund Weitzman was a 22-year-old medical school student at Temple University and looking for a good summer job. He was offered employment by the University of Pennsylvania test administrator and medical technician, Calvin Triol, and soon found himself in the midst of "a lot of commercial product testing" in the Philadelphia prisons.[19] By far, Sigmund Weitzman's "worst experience" that summer resulted from the application of a new "hair lotion" on the inmate volunteers. A few days after the experiment began, Weitzman was pinned against a wall by a 6'5", 250-pound, angry inmate. "I was scared to death. He threatened to kill me." The inmate was Roy Williams, serving a 9-to-23-month sentence. (Upon his release from prison, the soft-spoken Roy "Tiger" Williams would go on to establish a formidable 39-and-4 record in the ring, boxing against such heavyweights as Jimmy Young, Ernie Shavers, Ken Norton, and Larry Holmes.) He became enraged when he started losing his hair in large clumps after using Weitzman's test shampoo. Williams, too, remembers the test. "I didn't really have a dandruff problem, but I did after that test. The lotion removed my hair and anything else I had on my head."[20]

Sigmund Weitzman would go on to earn his medical degree and establish a solid career in medicine as a cancer researcher. "I saw some bizarre things," says Dr. Weitzman, reflecting on events that happened more than a quarter-century ago.[21] He says the many deodorants tested were "absolutely awful," and the athlete's foot treatment, in which liquid medication was placed between the inmates' toes, required an "incredible ability to withstand odor." A little over a decade later, he was shaken by newspaper revelations disclosing information indicating that the prison experiments were far more dangerous than he had ever suspected. As part of the University of Pennsylvania human experimentation program, Dr. Weitzman may have worked closely with several extremely dangerous substances—one of them, the potent carcinogen dioxin. The newspaper articles both frightened and angered him. He is still surprised that a scientist as eminent as Dr. Albert Kligman could have performed such experiments without informing the volunteers and staff members.

IV

One person with a unique vantage point is 73-year-old William McCafferty, currently at Graterford State Penitentiary. Blind in one eye and suffering from several physical ailments, McCafferty was imprisoned at Holmesburg between 1950 and 1955. He was present at the medical research program's founding in 1951–52 and witnessed its subsequent development.

A dependable worker, inmate McCafferty was given the job of running the prison commissary. The commissary job was one of the best an inmate could get and McCafferty said he "ate and smoked like hell," but he grew disenchanted because merchandise was stolen on a regular basis.[22] "A guy caught stealing was tops with the warden so they wouldn't get rid of him and they wouldn't let me hire good guys." Disgusted and frustrated, he finally asked a guard who ran the X-ray unit for a new job. Because he had been a "medic and a surgical technician in the Army" and was familiar with first aid procedures, he was assigned the job of doctors' clerk at ten cents a day. This new position offered perks, including pay seven days a week instead of five, and a private cell while everybody else was double-celled. McCafferty was especially happy about one additional perk: as the inmate nurse, he was the only inmate to receive a quart of fresh milk each day. Prisoners in the hospital shared 14 quarts and the other 1,200 prisoners had to suffer with the bland, powdered variety. Equally important, his cell was moved to H Block and rarely locked. On call 24 hours a day, it was his responsibility to respond to an inmate's illness—including those prisoners taking part in medical research for the University of Pennsylvania.

In the early years, according to McCafferty, patch tests were the only experiments that were performed on the inmates. "The shower room [exposing the distinctive scar tissue and skin discolorations] disclosed who was on the test," he says with a chuckle. Some of their experiments were "burning the hell out of the guys." By 1954 the university had expanded its facilities to include biopsies, soap studies, and investigations of skin and nail regeneration. The soap tests appeared fairly safe and simple according to McCafferty. The inmate volunteers would wash their hands in distilled water with a particular brand of soap and then rinse their hands in four separate basins of water.

Some experiments were far more offensive to the test subjects' hands. On one test, the university doctors proposed to extract one fingernail at $50 a piece from each of the six inmates. With the other inmates looking on, the doctors took the first volunteer, numbed his finger with Novocain, and placed his hand in a vice to immobilize the finger. But when the inmates saw the doctor grab a large pair of pliers and approach the volunteer, they panicked at the primitive methodology. Yelling "Hell no, not for fifty bucks," they refused to cooperate any further. A quick bargaining session yielded a three-fold increase in pay, "but the inmates were sorry when the Novocain wore off." "Two or three hours later that son-of-a-bitch really started to throb and hurt like hell." McCafferty believes the university doctors were interested in "the wound, [how a] manhandled finger reacted to abuse."

As the first aid man, McCafferty helped those who fell ill after the medical personnel had left. "At 4 P.M. that place closed up like a tomb. The guards came to my cell at 12, 2, 3 o'clock in the morning and woke me up saying 'Ken, Ken.' A guy was sick and I'd have to go to the blocks. I'd take his temperature, pulse, blood pressure, ask him questions, and try to find out what was wrong with him." McCafferty reported to the guard who called the doctor if he thought it was serious. McCafferty described the symptoms over the phone, and the doctor told him what to do. If medication was indicated, the guard went to the prison pharmacy and got the drugs. In an emergency, the doctor came to the prison, but this was rare.[23]

William McCafferty remembers one particular occasion when the doctors came in to handle an emergency and stayed for several days and nights. The university research unit was trying to find a preventative to poison ivy and had recruited a dozen inmates to participate in an experiment. "Six guys were given a special serum," and the other six, placebos. After receiving their injections, "four of the prisoners went back to the block and got sick [with an] immediate reaction…[they] went to the hospital in terrible shape." The two others passed out, one on the block, the other in the center control area of the prison rotunda—he "had no blood pressure." A doctor from the University of Pennsylvania Hospital arrived and "stayed with the patients for two days." The serum, according to McCafferty, was "examined at the lab and found to be a chemical that can have a dramatic impact on a person's blood pressure. It is now used in surgery to reduce blood pressure." After the doctors left, McCafferty took the "inmate's blood pressure each evening" to ensure that there were no relapses.[24]

The general public received a glowing, sanitized version of Dr. Albert Kligman's "scientific quest" through a full, two-page spread in *Life* magazine. Entitled "The Poison Ivy Picker of Pennypack Park," the 1955 article praised the dedication of a Philadelphia physician "crawling through the bushes" searching for "bouquets of poison ivy" for his Holmesburg experiments. "In 300 trials," the article stated, "only a dozen or so vaccinated volunteers have had more than a brief local rash."[25] The article led readers to believe the tests were "mild" and far from the traumatic experience witnessed by McCafferty and others inside the jail.

V

Despite such unnerving sights as prisoners fainting, being carried to the hospital, and sporting surgical bandages, according to McCafferty, the vast majority of the inmate population wanted to "get on the gravy train." "[In the fifties], minimum wage was real low, and $5 a test was decent."[26] The testing program was so desirable, in fact, that racial strife developed around it. Black prisoners protested that "only whites were on the tests, [they] get all the money and we don't get anything." Black prisoners were segregated on two of the ten cell blocks. By the time McCafferty left Holmesburg in 1955 to serve another five-year term at Graterford, black prisoners were housed on the E, F, and G Blocks with three to a cell, and their portion of the prison population was climbing toward 50 percent. The protest by African-American inmates was settled quickly when test administrators assured the prisoners that they did not discriminate and the tests were open to everyone. Nonetheless, accusations circulated for years that black inmates were directed to the less desirable tests with lower pay. According to McCafferty: "Back in those days, inmates did everything. They took the fingerprints of new arrivals, figured out the time an inmate would serve, classified prisoners, and cleaned the weapons [in the prison arsenal]....The guards only carried the keys and opened the cells."[27] These staff positions held true for the research program, and it is probable that the racism in American culture was reflected in the prison inmates' decisions about who participated in a given test.

According to various scholarly publications by Kligman during his Holmesburg years, experimental protocols occasionally required racial separation, with some experiments using exclusively white prisoners and others reserved for blacks. For example, one 1957 experiment designed "to promote the inoculation of human skin with...ectodermotropic viruses" such as "wart virus...herpes simplex and herpes zoster" was reserved for "healthy, colored, male volunteers" between the ages of 20 and 45 years of age.[28] Another, on "experimental inflammation and inflammatory dermatoses," targeted "10 healthy white subjects" who were paid to submerge one arm in a sodium lauryl sulfate solution one hour a day for 55 days in a row.[29]

As time went on and the number of tests multiplied, the research program required more careful organization; civilians assumed the staff positions formerly held by the inmates. Good-paying jobs for inmates dwindled, making the pay from the research program even more attractive and the inmate grapevine more important. Inmate workers, who had access to bits and pieces of information garnered by listening to doctors' conversations and surreptitiously reading office paperwork, were able to advise their friends about upcoming tests. As McCafferty says, "the head inmate-worker knew a lot."[30] Leodus Jones, a former drug abuser who spent most of the 1960s in Holmesburg, says, "I didn't like them at all." Unless he had been warned by an inmate worker who knew "what tests to get on and what tests to stay away from,...I just did them when necessary."[31] Matthew Epps, a Holmesburg inmate who did clerical work as an intake interviewer for the university program, says: "Guys were told you don't want to be on this test, but on that test."[32] "Inmates were advised" by other inmates or by friendly medical technicians who knew which experiments were desirable or undesirable. The message was clear: "Some tests were dangerous."[33]

Jay Biose spent the early 1970s in the Philadelphia prison system awaiting trial and the subsequent appeal of his murder conviction. He had a friend who had started work as a clerk/typist for the university's smaller satellite testing program at the Philadelphia Detention Center, and advised Biose to do the same. Biose remembers being told, "'[They] need more help down there'" and he should talk to them about getting a job.[34] His academic background impressed the administrators, and soon, Biose was placing "cotton swabs and tape" on the backs, shoulders, and arms of test subjects. Occasionally he handled "direct application of liquids and jelly" on the men, but mostly he was part of a "three-man team in an assembly-line process....[The technician] placed the chemical on the inmate, [I] placed tape [over the site], and another worker kept the books."

The three-man team made their rounds every day, usually in the early afternoon, and tried to visit the three cell blocks and four dormitories that made up the Detention Center. Biose says they "saw about 40 to 50 inmates" on their rounds, "at least five inmates per cell block." He saw many "prisoners that were burned by the tests," but he just passed it off as an "adverse reaction to some of the cosmetics" that were being tested.

He knew that many of the prisoners were wary of the experiments, but he also believes the inmates were streetwise enough to realize that you "don't get something for nothing"—the university testing program was "a con...[and] there were some risks." To temper the fear and doubt inmates had about particular tests, the medical technician suggested that Biose wear a false set of gauze patches and tape; the technician would pay him as though he were on the test. Biose cooperated and donned "dummy strips to deceive the inmates and convince them the tests were okay."

Other prison personnel would periodically try to steer the men away from the tests. Albert Levitt, for example, a senior psychologist for the Philadelphia Common Pleas Court, first began his long career in the criminal justice system when he entered Holmesburg Prison in 1962. He provided psychological testing and counseling to thousands of prisoners over the years and was able to observe the inmate experiments firsthand. He says "[the cosmetic tests] were causing all kinds of burns" and "the Army was running all kinds of tests. I told my guys in the group to stay away from those tests, but they didn't listen, and some went crazy from those LSD tests....I warned them, 'You don't know what you're being exposed to.'"[35]

Most institutional personnel, however, not only kept their doubts to themselves but also described the testing program as a valuable institutional resource. The prison system's few beleaguered social workers carried standard individual caseloads of 150 to 200 men. It became commonplace for social workers to suggest the University of Pennsylvania medical program as a likely source of income when regular prison jobs were unavailable. "If somebody didn't have money for commissary and wasn't on the list for a job, the social worker would say you can go to the U of P testing operation," says Priscilla Becroft, a Holmesburg social worker who started in 1972.[36] She adds, "The medical program was thought to be benign at the time." Tom Shouler, another social worker, says: "We only knew what we were told. It was a U of P program to test new cosmetics and perfumes. We never knew any more than that."[37]

Scott Willson, a prison social worker from 1970 to 1983, recalls, "Nobody really investigated what the tests were about. We questioned it among ourselves, but nobody looked into it. The medical personnel walked around in white coats and looked very official and authoritative."[38] Willson points out that the experiments also served the "jail culture...at Holmesburg; inmates liked it [because it was] the best money in the joint....Guards were happy because inmates [were] making money and causing fewer problems."

Former guards admit that the university's inmate experiments were viewed by some as a management tool. By keeping the inmates busy and supplying them with funds for commissary, it lessened tension in the jail among better-behaved prisoners. "I thought it would disrupt the prison," says retired Captain Alex Gougnin, but "I found it quite a help."[39] On occasion, he used the threat of terminating a prisoner's participation in a test as a stern warning to disruptive inmates. "'If you don't behave, we'll take you off the test,'" Gougnin recalls saying more than once. "For the inmates, it was a privilege to be on the testing program."

Captain Gougnin, now in his seventies, spent 25 years working in the Philadelphia Prison System before retiring in 1978. He can quickly recall a long list of inmate experiments that included the usual, "shave creams, mouthwashes, deodorants, and detergents," and the unusual, "women's lingerie and soda water." As with other guards who witnessed the unusual activity on Holmesburg's H Block, he recalled one eerie scene after another. He remembers "burn tests" that left bad scars "on their quadriceps muscles." The device used to burn the test subjects was referred to as a "ray gun" by the inmates. Gougnin says: "The burns went deep into the skin. I don't know how the inmates submitted to that." Gougnin periodically observed the doctors applying various salves to the burns. He remembers inmates walking around with devices designed to collect skin and perspiration, "1–1½-inch stainless steel cups strapped to their foreheads." He recalls "scalp transplants," unsuccessful attempts to rejuvenate hair growth by moving an inmate's "hair from the back of the scalp to the front." The experiment that left a particularly strong impression on Captain Gougnin was one that nearly resulted in the deaths of seven inmates. He believes the experiment involved liver biopsies, which he claims had begun in the early 1960s and were quite common on H Block. But one weekend "seven patients almost expired" and everyone was in a "panic" when the university doctors could not be located. Because of such emergencies, Gougnin believed then that the program should be discontinued, or, at the very least, that the inmates "should be paid more" for their participation.

The University of Pennsylvania testing program continued to grow as the years passed, and correctional officers such as Gougnin saw a steady increase in medical staff, experiments, and scientific apparatus. The research program "started as a trickle and then went full force in the early 1960s," says Gougnin. He remembers that the H Block lab held an array of sophisticated equipment such as a

Coulter Counter; a machine that performed rapid blood analysis which was so state-of-the-art that even nearby "Abington Hospital didn't have it."

Most hospitals also did not have three trailers, modified to include padded cells and high-tech monitoring equipment. In the mid-1960s, the Army initiated new and secret mind-control experiments that required special facilities. Three trailers were brought inside the prison walls and placed alongside H Block in the prison yard. It was an unprecedented addition to the old institution and a source of tremendous dread and speculation. "It was the first time I saw padded cells" recalls Gougnin. Rumors were widespread throughout the jail and the whole process, the secrecy and precedence given the administrators, made Gougnin very uncomfortable. He asks now in exasperation, "Who gave them the power to take over the prison?"

Most inmates, looking for a way to earn money, were less critical. Withers Ponton, who went through so many scarring biopsies, is matter-of-fact about it: "Hell, I needed the money. Every day I went over to H Block to see if they could use me." For Ponton and many others, money was not just *a* factor, it was the *sole* factor. In fact, of the dozens of former Holmesburg Prison inmates who took part in the experiments that I was able to locate and interview, everyone mentioned the need for money as the reason—the only reason—they took part in the medical tests.

Rick Mancini, now in his fifties, is a prime example. Serving 15 months in the county jail in the mid-1960s, Mancini "didn't worry" about possible test repercussions; he "needed the money."[40] He remembers participating in "three or four tests" that included a "pill test, biopsy test, and toothpaste test" and does not hesitate to show the scars on his forearm and back from the biopsies. Mancini says he "didn't get paid very much, about $25, but it was a lot of money back then." Nearly 30 years later, he says: "I wouldn't do it now, I know better. As you get older you get wiser."

George Porter tells the same story. Arrested for armed robbery at age 26 in 1967, he spent a year at Holmesburg awaiting trial. Porter "needed money badly at the time and [was told] you could earn some money at the U of P studies."[41] He went through a series of

"30-day patch tests" and was exposed to several "creams and dyes" that caused a lot of "itching and irritation." Porter recalls "some guys passing out" and requiring hospitalization, but says, "I had no problem with the tests, I needed the money." He estimates he made between $400 and $500 during his year at Holmesburg.

Andy Hollick, now 46 years old, says in retrospect, "the pay was bad, but it was the only thing in the prison."[42] Soon after his arrival at Holmesburg, Hollick "participated in several patch tests and one diet test." One of the experiments "placed a certain medication" on his forehead that discolored his skin. The problem required extra treatment by "doctors to regain the true color." He says, "Guys were paid $100 and $200 for a seven- or eight-week test." James Lewis, a lifer at Graterford who spent nine months at Holmesburg in 1965, says much the same. "It wasn't big money, but they paid you."[43]

According to several national studies on the subject of human experimentation in penal facilities, other reasons given by inmates for volunteering for such experiments, apart from money, were: the expectation of better food, cleaner and more comfortable living quarters, patriotic or altruistic feelings, a desire to aid scientific discovery, a brief reprieve from the terminal boredom or threats of violence on the cell block, and the hope of a sentence reduction.[44]

One study showed that over 50 percent of the prisoners claimed a desire for better living conditions. Some, who were ill-at-ease in the institution or "loners," gravitated toward the medical researchers as "the only group that would take them."[45] The vast majority of prisoner comments, particularly among those serving time in state or federal institutions, cite early release as the central motivating factor.

At Holmesburg Prison, however, the prisoners I spoke with said they did not volunteer for various experiments because they were bored, patriotic, or wanted better housing. They needed money and the university research program paid the most. Not one of the many former prisoners interviewed mentioned any reason other than money as the prime motivation for participating in such experiments. Indeed, interviewees scoff at the suggestion that some of their brethren in the tests might have been motivated by patriotism or the advance of science. "No inmate volunteered for patriotic reasons," snickers Billy Allison. "They did it for the money, pure and simple."[46] Al Zabala is equally disdainful. "No one took tests for patriotic duty or because they were good people. They were doing it for financial gain."[47]

Those few inmates who saw in the Holmesburg testing experience the opportunity to live better on H Block or to contribute to society, still emphasize payment as central to their participation. Darren Sellner spent nearly ten months in Holmesburg in the late sixties, and would "harass doctors on H Block" to get on the test projects.[48] He speaks of the "sense of self-worth" and the "exceptionally clean" and "professionally run" research unit. "It was a very beneficial program for the inmates," says Sellner. "It gave them money so they didn't have to wheel and deal for things." He says he had "no hesitancy at all" about participating, and "was really upset when [he] read they were discontinuing the tests. They were destroying another opportunity for the inmates." The money he earned in the Holmesburg experiments would have been "really helpful" to him when he left the prison, if he hadn't squandered it when he was released. "I had over $200, but I used it for drugs instead," he says.

Cash greased the wheels of the university research program. As Fred Foxworth, a retired deputy warden says, "They never had a problem getting volunteers. The inmates needed the money."[49] Jack Lopinson, a Graterford lifer who witnessed many of the Holmesburg experiments in the mid-1960s says, "The biggest reason guys went into the [research program was that] drug tests were the best-paying jobs. Prison [labor] didn't pay and here was easy money. Guys had no source of money" independent of what the prison system offered.[50]

"As many as could get a test would," claims retired officer Hank Brame. "It was more money than a prisoner had ever seen before. For a two-week test, a guy could make $100."[51] By participating in as many tests as possible, some inmates, especially those with less severe charges and low bail, could raise the 10 percent bail bond required for freedom. On several occasions I contributed $10 or $20 to inmates who had successfully petitioned the courts to reduce their bail and were trying to raise the necessary funds from guards, social workers, and teachers with whom they were friendly. The majority of inmates in the Philadelphia prison system in the late 1960s and early 1970s were unsentenced prisoners awaiting trial. Money to hire an attorney or make bail before a forthcoming trial was a constant preoccupation among these inmates.

Another preoccupation was the commissary. Prisons are stark, barren environments that can be made slightly more palatable with weekly purchases of cookies, cakes, candy, cigarettes, and personal items at the prison commissary. "Holmesburg was a pigsty back then," recalls Al Butler, "and commissary meant a lot. There were no jobs…and the men were idle. But survival was important." Butler became the program's official photographer. "Kligman okayed me to be the [research program's] photographer and paid me $25 a month" to photograph inmates with interesting medical problems. He says, "A few times a week" any inmate who seemed to have a "severe reaction" to a test such as rashes from "detergent tests" would be brought to him to capture on film the "progress of the rash." "Everything was done as cheaply as they could. They were just preying on people. Using an inmate was cheaper than buying a chimpanzee and the results were better." In the end it was an "economic decision."[52]

This was especially true for prisoners who were charged with high-profile capital-felony cases and could expect to be interned at least a year or two at Holmesburg before their trial. Ron Keenan, for example, stayed away from the experiments for the first six months of his incarceration, but then submitted because he "needed money for commissary."[53] During the next two years, Keenan became a regular subject for a cross-section of research projects, many of which he did not understand. "I got a needle in my spine for $7," says Keenan matter-of-factly. "They put a chemical in, but for some reason it didn't work," and the experiment was canceled. In one "pill test" designed to "quicken the sun tanning process," Keenan doubled up in pain with "cramps you wouldn't believe" after swallowing four pills on H Block. They explained to him that this "was something new coming on the market" and he would have to go in "the exercise yard for 20 minutes every day for a week or two" in order to capture the sun's rays. Keenan doesn't recall if he developed a tan, but "the terrible stomach cramps" are still hard to forget. Although he was open to most experiments, there were some he wanted no part of. "I heard about the Army test from other guys and I said 'I don't want any of that stuff.'" He claims he was "told they were LSD tests," and says that after seeing a number of inmates return from the trailers he didn't doubt it.

Some inmates, while they needed money, had no intention of participating in the tests. Most of them were either frightened by the specter of subjecting their bodies to unknown consequences or opposed them for religious reasons. In the opinion of some non-test takers, those who participated were fools. Al Butler, for instance, argues that he never underwent any tests because "I've got more...brains."[54] He says the inmates who volunteered "were assholes, illiterate, and [had no] money for commissary." Allan Lawson, now 59 years old, first entered prison in 1960 on a robbery charge and would spend the next decade in and out of jail, but would never succumb to the temptations of the research program. One of his strongest recollections of an initial stint inside Eastern State Penitentiary was "the guys in the showers...who had all these scars and discolorations on their skin."[55] When he asked what had happened to them, he heard about the Holmesburg experiments. In time, Lawson learned the tests were the only way "guys could make money in jail" and some were coming out with several thousand dollars on the books. But he says: "I swore to myself that 'I'd never get on one of those tests.' I didn't need money that bad."

Raymond Crawford, now 49 years old and in the 27th year of a life sentence, says, "Everyone did it for money. There was a small number of jobs in the county jail and men needed money."[56] But Crawford felt the university "people were taking advantage of a bad situation." "We didn't know anything about what they were testing" or how the "things you would ingest," would affect subjects years later. "It just wasn't worth the chance."

Simon Khaadim Ahad, another lifer and now in his fifties, rejected the opportunity to participate in the experiments for religious reasons. A former member of the Nation of Islam, Ahad says the

"Muslims had taken a position opposed to the tests" and were not cooperative when U of P test recruiters came over to D Block, where most of the Muslims were housed, "to try and solicit guinea pigs."[57] Ahad remembers them "coming around on the blocks with a cart of testing material." "We told the doctors, 'Absolutely not' because of religious beliefs. We knew white men were devils, and the tests were dangerous." He knows that "some brothers submitted for economic reasons," but maintains that very few devout Muslims agreed to participate.

Almost all inmates agree, however, that those who did succumb to the doctors' overtures had very little idea, if any, of what ingredient, solution, chemical, or drug they were actually testing. Most important, the majority of men claim to have never heard the words, "informed consent," much less understood the concept's importance. Their economic needs and ignorance, combined with the medical community's cavalier approach, produced a program on the edge of medical ethics. All of the former test subjects agree that, as Al Zabala says: "Inmates were never told the truth about what they were being exposed to. If you had a complication they told you not to go to the regular prison doctors, but to see the test technicians. They were reluctant to have outside doctors involved."[58] Thomas Sims remembers that he signed release forms, but was "never told what chemicals they were giving [him]."[59] Withers Ponton says he signed a release acknowledging payment and listing next of kin, but the release did not describe "what [he was] testing or being exposed to."[60] Veteran test-taker, Keenan says the test-givers "never explained that there would be any discomfort from the patch test," but the "blisters made it very uncomfortable to lie on his back."[61] Many of the men were left with blistered and scarred torsos. The whole ordeal was "quite painful" he admits, but "I needed the money."

Prison staff are equally skeptical about how informed the test subjects were before they gave their consent. Retired Captain Alex Gougnin says: "The inmates did not know what they were being exposed to. [Test administrators] didn't tell the inmates" what the tests were about or how they could affect them the next day, month, or years in the future.[62] The former superintendent of prisons,

Edmund Lyons, has the same opinion. "The tests were always represented to be quite innocent and beneficial."[63] Furthermore, he claims that the inmates, many of whom could not read, and most of whom "had about a third-grade level of reading comprehension,...couldn't understand the consent forms." And they received little advice from the prison staff since, as Lyons believes, the people at highest levels in the prison hierarchy shared a belief in the innocuous nature of the tests.

Dr. Sigmund Weitzman says that the "releases inmates had to sign" could be technical—some included "liver function measures."[64] "I couldn't even understand them," says Weitzman. "How would an uneducated inmate?" According to his recollection: "Inmates were never told the substance" they were being exposed to; they were told only that it was a "commercial product" being tested "for sensitivity—not toxicity." This language cannot have fully informed an imprisoned population made up primarily of functional illiterates and high school dropouts. In the end, however, a combination of economic distress, physical imprisonment, and a naive faith that they would not be harmed brought many Holmesburg inmates to the research lab.

But questions remain. The thousands of incarcerated and economically desperate men who took part in patch tests have most likely spent years wondering about the creams that were spread across their faces, backs, and arms. The many who underwent skin biopsies have questioned whether the needles they received just prior to excising the skin were filled with harmless colored dyes or more ominous fluids containing radioactive isotopes. And finally, the men who ventured into the feared Army trailers have wondered whether it was really LSD that caused such bizarre and frightening visions or an even more powerful stimulant that may be affecting them still.

For society too, questions linger. How could the Holmesburg experiments have proceeded over the course of three decades without government officials, investigative journalists, and relatives of the test subjects becoming more alarmed? And why did physician-researchers and the medical community in general—a revered profession morally obligated to uphold the Hippocratic Oath and the Nuremberg Code—allow callous research practices to continue for so long?

Two

"It Was Like a Farmer Seeing a Fertile Field."

I

Holmesburg Prison was more than a half century old when the first experiments on humans were conducted behind its massive front doors. Holmesburg had already left its mark on Philadelphia, especially on the thousands of troubled, violent men who had been imprisoned there. When it closed nearly 100 years after its opening, Holmesburg had well earned its reputation for bloodshed and brutality.

The structure was built at a cost of $1.4 million and was designed to be "the embodiment of the most enlightened application" of penal philosophy in the state.[1] But the day it opened to prisoners in 1896, one reporter described the 17-acre facility as sending the harsh and unforgiving message: "Abandon hope all ye who enter here." Another newspaper man mused on the facility's opening: "Not a window can be seen, and a spectator gathers the impression that light, too, is denied the unfortunate who are condemned to spend years of seclusion without these abhorrent limits."[2] A forbidding fieldstone wall surrounded the prison: 35 feet high and 8 feet wide at its base, it narrowed to 3 feet at the capstone—an impregnable sheet of solid stone.

Within, the Holmesburg architecture followed the classic spoke-and-wheel design popularized by Eastern State Penitentiary in the 1820s: ten cell blocks radiating out from a central hub or rotunda. The cell blocks were constructed in varying lengths, some containing 68 cells, some 74, and others 78. Each cell was 6 feet by 8 feet, huge by contemporary standards. Although the cells were designed to hold one inmate, Philadelphia soon found that number a luxury:

the cells usually housed two men, and on occasion as many as five. Initially, inmates were to be "prisoners under sentence," but in fact, by the end of the Holmesburg Prison medical experiments in the mid-1970s, the majority of inmates were unsentenced prisoners awaiting trial.

During its first 50 years of operation, Holmesburg hosted numerous bloody riots, clever escapes, and violent encounters between guards and inmates. Rigid rules and regulations were vigorously enforced, "dark cells" or punishment cells had been created "to control the prisoners," and nearly "half the prisoners [were] employed at some useful labor."[3] Visitors were struck by the prison's "odor." "It is the scent of hundreds of men mingled with the smell of disinfectants. Keepers do not notice it, but it is heavy and ominous, and is probably the same that gives warning to startled wild animals that pick up the scent of a hunter down the wind."

Holmesburg prisoners quickly earned a reputation for "toughness and hardness."[4] In the aftermath of a bloody riot in 1929, prison wardens from several different county and state facilities canceled plans to temporarily accept Holmesburg inmates. Those few county wardens who already had accepted inmates sent them back after they "started trouble" and proved "too tough" for the smaller institutions to handle. One upstate warden complained about the Philadelphia prisoners' "hardness" and expressed fear that his institution would be "corrupted" by their presence. Replied John Bennett, then deputy superintendent of Holmesburg: "We didn't transfer our worst men by any means. We purposely kept the leaders and agitators here with us, but now it looks as if all the prisons are going to dump the men back on us...the other prisons don't seem to like our men at all."

The inmates, themselves, had horrendous stories to tell. In 1929, Harold Hubbs, a 28-year-old former Camden policeman serving a "60-day sentence for violation of the dry laws," faced amputation of his feet after prison injuries had gone unattended.[5] His legs had been broken and, Hubbs said, "they threw me into my cell, and I pleaded for a hot-water bottle...to bathe them in, but it was not forthcoming."

Though prisoners said brutal living conditions were commonplace, Holmesburg overseers were rarely reprimanded for excessive discipline. But there were exceptions. In 1929, Charles Sorber, a tyrannical deputy superintendent with 33 years of experience, was sought by authorities when he fled after the discovery that he had flogged prisoners on a regular basis. Apparently he assigned the "three Musketeers, a group of colored convicts" to "welcome new prisoners" to the institution.[6] According to the city district attorney, Sorber would give the three men "small favors" and "additional rations of tobacco" to enter "the cells of new inmates and beat them."

For inmates who challenged prison authority, life could be hell. A particularly ugly incident occurred in August 1938, during an inmate food strike. Determined to break the strike and punish the ringleaders, the authorities escorted nearly two dozen prisoners to "the Klondike," a punishment unit housed in a separate corner of the prison yard. The small brick building contained few cells, but had a bank of radiators generating incredible heat. After an unusually hot August weekend in the Klondike with the windows shut tight and the radiators turned on full blast, the strike was over. And so were the lives of four inmates—cooked to death in a simulated oven. Survivors told a horrifying story that captured national attention and generated newspaper headlines in Philadelphia for months to come. After visiting the site, a shaken Pennsylvania Governor George Earle of Pennsylvania called the prison "a torture chamber," the perpetrators "the cruelest sadists who ever lived," and set about to ensure that such acts could never happen again in a Pennsylvania prison.[7] Several guards and high-ranking prison administrators were indicted, tried, and convicted. The "Bake-Oven Deaths" at Holmesburg were soon forgotten except for inside the walls of the old jail, where the memory lingered as a warning to troublesome prisoners.

By the postwar period and the introduction of a medical program dependent on human experimentation, Holmesburg had changed very little; a predatory atmosphere engulfed the institution, food was bad, jobs were few, and there were still 720 manually operated cells in a maximum-security facility that now held from 1,000 to 1,400 tense prisoners.

The city's prison system included two other jails, the House of Correction and the Philadelphia Detention Center, both built along the banks of Pennypack Creek, a stone's throw from Holmesburg.

The older facility, the House of Correction, went back decades and was also built in the traditional 19th-century radial design. Referred to as "The Creek" by both guards and inmates, the House of Correction was a medium-security facility that was designed for "drunks, vagrants, and women misdemeanants." As the years passed, these lesser offenders had been replaced by more aggressive adult and juvenile offenders. The population of the facility fluctuated, but during the early 1950s, when the medical experiments began, the average daily population was approximately 800, and would climb to 1,100 inmates through most of the mid- and late 1960s.

The newest facility was the Philadelphia Detention Center, opened in 1963 to replace Moyamensing, the old municipal prison built in 1835 at 10th and Reed Streets in south Philadelphia. "D.C.," as it was commonly called, was a modern and state-of-the-art penal facility. Departing from the radial design, the prison contained three cell blocks and four dormitories, and usually held between 700 and 1,000 prisoners. The detention center became the system's receiving prison and classification center, holding inmates anywhere from a day to years depending upon the charge, bail level, or security risk. Generally, half the population turned over every two weeks as prisoners were shipped off to "The Burg" or The Creek and new inmates entered the system. Holmesburg remained the beast of the city's correctional system: an American gulag reserved for the worst of the worst.

II

Medical research under Dr. Albert Kligman began in the county penal system in the early 1950s, when Holmesburg Prison was suffering from another outbreak of athlete's foot, a malady common to a large, unsanitary, residential facility. Many of the 1,200 prisoners had been diagnosed with the fungus infection and the institution's small, beleaguered medical staff was searching for the best treatment. The prison pharmacist came across an article written by Albert M. Kligman, professor of dermatology at the University of Pennsylvania Medical School, and called the author.

Dr. Kligman completed his formal education in Pennsylvania, and—through his many students, publications, and patented discoveries—had developed a worldwide reputation. Born on March 17, 1916, in Philadelphia, and educated in the Philadelphia public school system, Albert M. Kligman became a Phi Beta Kappa graduate of Pennsylvania State College in 1939, and by 1947 acquired both a Ph.D. and M.D. from the University of Pennsylvania. Kligman came from humble surroundings and was able to complete his undergraduate career only with the financial assistance of Simon Greenberg, a local rabbi who took an interest in the precocious student.

A prolific author, Kligman wrote scores of medical articles on a variety of dermatological subjects. His earliest works, written in the early 1940s, before he entered medical school, concentrated on the mushroom. According to Dr. Leon Kneebone,[8] a noted mushroom expert and Pennsylvania State University professor, Kligman was the author of a respected "handbook on mushroom culture [that was] widely used in the 1950s, 1960s, and 1970s."[9] And one of his papers dealing with the "genetics of commercial mushrooms is still quoted."[10] As Kneebone aptly phrases it, Kligman "left edible fungi work to go to medical school and specialize in human fungi."[11] This unusual interest stemmed from the fact that Kligman had received his doctorate in botany (mycology), specializing in the study of fungus. He told one newspaper reporter that he had "planned to go on a government-sponsored botany expedition to South America during World War II, [but] when it was learned that, as a youth, he had entertained communist sympathies, his trip was canceled." "'It's true, what can I say?' Kligman said. 'Youth is stupid.'"[12] Rejected by both the Army and Navy because of a recurring pilonidal cyst, he followed the advice of his first wife, Beatrice Troyan, entered medical school, and graduated at age 31.[13] He chose his specialty at the University of Pennsylvania after it was suggested to him that his knowledge of fungus offered a natural start to a career in dermatology.

After medical school, Kligman continued to pursue his interest in fungi. His studies centered on the various human fungus infections currently plaguing the American populace, and he published numerous scientific papers on the subject: "Improved Technique for Diagnosing Ringworm Infections and Moniliasis," "The Hotchkiss-McManus Stain for the Histopathologic Diagnosis of Fungus Disease," and "Application of Potassium Hydroxide to the

Skin as an Aid in Direct Examination of Scales for Fungi"—the articles that sparked the call from Holmesburg.[14] During the 1940s,
microsporum audouini, for example, an organism that causes scalp
ringworm, had grown to epidemic proportions in most major U.S.
cities. In an attempt to "critically" evaluate "the real value" of new
therapies to combat the troubling affliction, Kligman published a
paper in 1951 that described a "controlled experiment" that "experimentally infected" retarded children in order to test various
fungistatic preparations.[15] In a study of ringworm (tinea capitis) that
was published in a leading dermatology journal, Kligman wrote:

> The data reported in this paper derive from observations on exper-
> imentally infected humans. The work was carried out at a state
> institution for congenital mental defectives where tinea capitis was
> endemic and the inmates subject to constant opportunity for infec-
> tion. The experimental circumstances were ideal in that a large
> number of individuals living under confined circumstances could
> be inoculated at will and the course of the disease minutely studied
> from its very onset. Biopsy material was freely available.[16]

Originally presented in 1951 at the 12th annual meeting of the
Society for Investigative Dermatologists, Kligman's address not only
escaped condemnation for cavalierly exploiting the most vulnerable
of institutionalized populations but also received praise for selecting
an "ideal," that is human, test population. The appreciative reviewer commented: "We have not been alive enough to the wealth of test
material that there is in penitentiaries, and the administrative officers are glad to have doctors work in their institutions. It indicates
that special attention is being paid to the welfare of their charges
and the inmates really enjoy it."[17]

The reviewer who so thoroughly endorsed Kligman's presentation and methodology was one of the most respected men in the
field, Dr. Frederick Deforest Weidman. An eminent researcher of
national reputation with decades of acclaimed experience, Dr.
Weidman was Emeritus Professor of Research in Dermatology and
Mycology at the University of Pennsylvania. A former president of
the American Dermatological Association and vice president of the
American Board of Dermatology and Syphilology, his views and
pronouncements carried great weight. The same issue of the *Journal*

of Investigative Dermatology that published Kligman's ringworm study was a "Festschrift Number" honoring Dr. Weidman. In a four-page testimonial, Dr. Donald Pillsbury described Weidman as exerting "an extraordinarily healthy and stimulating influence upon American dermatologists, both young and old, and [being]...a source of comfort to the many who have long depended upon him for advice and guidance....Moreover his guidance has always been exerted in a spirit of basic kindliness, and this is the hallmark of a great person."[18]

Though blessed with these extraordinary qualities and accomplishments, Weidman was unable to see the potential for damage to vulnerable individuals used as research material. In applauding such practices as "ideal," and encouraging physicians to use "the wealth of test material" in penitentiaries, Weidman was abandoning the principles of the recently enunciated Nuremberg Code. It is not surprising that an ambitious young physician like Albert Kligman became persuaded that state-of-the-art research required human test subjects, and that the use of institutionalized populations was perfectly acceptable.

The cavalier attitude toward using institutionalized groups as research subjects was so ingrained at the University of Pennsylvania Medical School (or, at the very least, in the dermatology department) that faculty members could openly describe such practices and make jokes about them in class lectures. Not surprisingly, Dr. Kligman, one of the department's most accomplished raconteurs, was at the center of these informative, and sometimes insensitive, lectures. According to a colleague, Dr. Kligman would describe how he "encouraged the development of ringworm by rubbing it in" the abraded scalp of retarded children.[19] Kligman would delight an audience of medical students and residents-in-training by telling them: "These kids want attention so bad, if you hit them over the head with a hammer they would love you for it."[20] After his success working with retarded children, it is understandable that Dr. Kligman quickly and easily adapted to the use of prison inmates as research material. In 1956, Dr. Kligman evidently combined retarded children and prisoners in the same study. He received a research grant of $13,949 from the Public Health Service, National Institutes of

Health, to examine "Pathologic Reactions of the Fingernails Including Fungus Infections."[21] The study was designed to "define the normal anatomy of the nail organ...to examine the pathologic responses of this organ to various experimental stresses as well as in spontaneously occurring disease states...to formulate the basic principles of a histopathology of the nails...[and] specifically investigate the pathogenesis of ringworm of the nails through the study of experimentally induced and naturally occurring infections."[22] Kligman listed two classes of subjects: individuals (to be found in hospitals and clinics) with spontaneous nail disease; and human volunteers (prisoners) in the Philadelphia County Prison, who "for a modest fee provide us with ideal opportunities." Kligman planned to take "punch biopsies from various portions of the nail folds, the nail matrix and the nail bed to determine the subsequent effects on growth and recuperation....In addition to removing portions of the nail organ surgically, we shall study the effects of applying caustic agents (silver nitrate, pheno)." Dr. Kligman claimed, "Work on fingernails has been almost non-existent because of the obvious difficulties in obtaining biopsy specimens....But in a preliminary survey we have convinced ourselves that the nail organ is a hardier structure than previously supposed and will tolerate a good deal of insult without permanent disability." Confidently, Kligman proceeded to use X-rays and a host of fungi on the test subjects.

As part of the budget for this project, the application listed "Human Subjects: 300 subjects (prisoners)—average rate $15.00 per subject" for a total of $4,500.00. Curiously, the budget section "expenditures for travel" includes 29 specific travel charges to Woodbine and Vineland, New Jersey.[23] In the rural portion of southern New Jersey, Woodbine (boys) and Vineland (girls) are the sites of large institutions for the mentally retarded and developmentally disabled. Kligman's medical assistants were traveling to the remote institutions on a regular basis, at least once and sometimes as often as four times a month. Although no specific mention is made in the application, retarded children were apparently part of the study that ran from September 1, 1956, to August 31, 1957.

III

The Holmesburg pharmacist who called Dr. Kligman about the athlete's foot epidemic asked him to visit the prison. Kligman agreed to come. "I went to the institution at their request," said Kligman in a 1995 interview.[24] "They had some very bad cases of athlete's foot in the institution." The exact year of his visit is unclear, but in a 1986 history of the dermatology program at the University of Pennsylvania, Dr. Kligman identified 1951 as the year he "received a call from Holmesburg Prison," shortly after he had "discovered the PAS stain for visualizing fungi."[25]

When Dr. Kligman entered the aging prison he was awed by the potential it held for his research. In 1966, he recalled in a newspaper interview: "All I saw before me were acres of skin. It was like a farmer seeing a fertile field for the first time."[26] The hundreds of inmates walking aimlessly before him represented a unique opportunity for unlimited and undisturbed medical research. He described it in this interview as "'an anthropoid colony, mainly healthy' under perfect control conditions."

As he told colleagues years later, "I began to go to the prison regularly, although I had no authorization. It was years before the authorities knew that I was conducting various studies on prisoner volunteers. Things were simpler then. Informed consent was unheard of. No one asked me what I was doing. It was a wonderful time."[27]

Kligman met with the superintendent, Frederick S. Baldi, whom years later Kligman recalls as "a rather tough man." Baldi was a physician who had worked at Holmesburg for a number of years before he was promoted to the top administrative position in the aftermath of the 1938 "Bake-Oven Deaths." Considering Baldi's medical experience and the postwar drive toward scientific advancement, it is not surprising that Dr. Kligman was granted his request to use prisoners for a series of dermatological experiments. Baldi retired in 1954, and Edward J. Hendrick, a tall, stern public official with strong religious beliefs, assumed command. He, too, believed the relationship could benefit both the prison and the medical community, and readily agreed to the professor's continued medical research in the prison. There were "no official contracts [between the University of Pennsylvania and] the prisons or city," Kligman said.[28] "The superintendent was strongly in favor of the program" and that's all that was needed. "I always had pleasant relations with Superintendent Hendrick. He was a very fine man."

A prison population provided a "natural" laboratory, recalls Dr. Kligman. The inmates were an "experimental population [he] could control." In a newspaper interview in 1960, the doctor said: "We know where they are, what they're doing, what they're eating; and if they're given pills six times a day, we know they are taken."[29] Such control over so many people—not to mention the commercial implications for dermatology—must have been intoxicating.

In a lengthy 1966 newspaper article about the origins and development of the Holmesburg Prison medical experimentation program, Dr. Kligman articulated his thoughts. "We had an ethical problem," the doctor admitted at one point. "How much right do you have to cause risk to a prisoner in medical tests from which he has no direct benefit? The tradition has been from ethical or moral considerations, to test only these people who could draw some direct benefit from the testing." The Holmesburg experience parted company with this tradition. Kligman said, "All the prisoner taking part in a test has is money. We pay him to lend us his body for some time. But we pre-determine whether a test is dangerous, and the prisoner has to depend on our judgment."[30]

In the same newspaper article, Superintendent Hendrick assured readers that "we will not approve anything like injecting live cancer cells. We will not approve anything which, on the face of it, would be deleterious to the physical well-being of an individual." The article went on to state that the prisoner volunteers were divided into two groups: a large group of more than 800 men who were used in the experiments, and a small unit of about three dozen men who acted as inmate technicians, assisted the doctors, and were taught to do the laboratory experiments. Kligman said, "We can teach our guys to become better technicians than any woman on the outside. A prisoner/technician isn't going anywhere while he is in prison. He may be a ragamuffin on the outside, but in two months we can make a highly skilled technician out of him."

Dr. Kligman held an equally paternalistic view of the test subjects. He describes an experiment testing anti-obesity drugs.

> A prison is the right place for such a test. [The men were confined
> in one room for six months.] How can you do a test like this on
> the outside—limiting a person to five grams of fat a day? We fed
> these men a milk-like emulsion. For six long months they had to
> take this lousy fluid. Now eating is one of the major pleasures of
> life. Suddenly you take all taste away from the men. They had all
> kinds of dreams…fantasies. Most of them became resigned and
> eventually came to like their diet. They reached a sensory vacuum.
> Meals meant nothing to them. But one guy couldn't take it after
> five months. Somewhere he got an onion and ate it. For him it was
> a paradisiacal experience after drinking that awful stuff. We dis-
> covered it and refused to pay him because the onion ruined the
> value of his test. Just one lousy onion deprived him of his money.
> He became violent. But we had to keep discipline. The man was
> just beside himself with rage.[31]

Dr. Kligman went on to discuss what the article termed his
"humanitarian" stance toward the prisoners.

> Many of the prisoners, for the first time in their lives, find them-
> selves in the role of important human beings. We say to them,
> "You're important, we need you."
> Once this is established, these guys will knock their brains out
> to please you. If the experiment does not pan out, they get
> depressed. They become emotionally involved in the project.
> The capacity to respond to love is greater than most people
> realize. I feel almost like a scoundrel—like Machiavelli—because
> of what I can do to them.[32]

For many years, it has been virtually impossible to find anyone
in either the prison system or the city administration knowledgeable about the Holmesburg experiments. Written records are sparse
because city officials did not supervise Dr. Kligman's research program. The difficulty of developing a comprehensive historical
account is compounded by Kligman's destruction of all his experimental data shortly after the research program closed in 1974.
Documentation emerges, however, in Kligman's own published articles and through the use of the Freedom of Information Act for government records. Less controversial than some of his more provocative

outside contract work, the published accounts of his dermatological studies can still provoke alarm at the cavalier use of inmates for risky experiments and the healing/harming paradox of the Holmesburg research program. For example:

1. A 1958 study inoculated scores of prisoners with such ectodermotropic viruses as wart virus, vaccinia, herpes simplex, and herpes zoster. The subjects of these experiments were "healthy colored male volunteers, 20 to 45 years of age" who volunteered to be "inoculated" several times. In the wart virus section of the study, "47 inoculations were performed in 7 volunteers in different skin areas (forearm, palm,...back, face, scalp,...and penis). All of the recipients developed at least one lesion, some of them two lesions at different localizations."[33]

2. In a 1957 study that examined "many different means of producing experimental infection" (ringworm) of the feet, Dr. Kligman applied "enormous quantities of fungi" to dozens of inmates. Some were made to wear boots "continually" for a week after being experimentally infected. Kligman commented that the "experimental advantages" of a "prison population" caused him to have a "fresh appreciation" for the disease.[34]

3. A 1961 study involving over 1,000 innoculations of "150 white and Negro subjects...21 to 65 years of age" with cutaneous moniliasis, a skin condition that can cause "pain and burning [and] when the inoculation area is large,...incapacitating lymphangitis....The subject may become sick and discomforted."[35]

4. Between 1965 and 1971, numerous other experiments infected prisoners with bacteria staphylococcus aureus,[36] candida albicans,[37] and melanocytes,[38] and exposed them to phototoxic drugs,[39] and long ultraviolet rays.[40]

IV

Kligman's research assistants based at the prison were in awe of him; the prison officials were dazzled; and medical students and residents who worked on projects at the prison were mesmerized—at least at first. Calvin Triol, who was hired away from a pharmaceutical company by the University of Pennsylvania in 1964 to assist Kligman with the prison experiments, calls him "the most brilliant man I have ever met."[41] Kligman was just "exploding with ideas" but, Triol adds, "not a good researcher in a pure sense." According to Triol, if preliminary research supported his expectations, he stopped the experiment ahead of schedule and assumed an outcome that had not yet been proved. Kligman had already moved on to "new ideas" and additional experiments.

Edmund Lyons, a former superintendent of the Philadelphia prison system and a warden during the height of Kligman's prison experiments in the 1960s, agrees with Triol about Kligman's superior intellectual prowess. "He was fascinating," says Lyons.[42] Alan Katz, hired by the University of Pennsylvania in the early 1960s as a pharmacist for the prison testing project, says, "He was a real enigma...a brilliant man."[43]

Kligman's peers and students in the medical profession were also impressed, although a few saw blemishes. For Clarence Livingood and Walter Shelley, two giants in the field of dermatological medicine with more than a century of combined service as physicians and department chairmen, Kligman is unique. "The man is a genius," says Dr. Livingood. "He's had tremendous accomplishments in his career."[44] Dr. Shelley calls Kligman an "absolutely unique individual" who was a "great teacher,...stellar lecturer," and a major force "on the cutting edge" of the profession.[45] Dr. Fred Urbach, Temple University's dermatology department chair for over three decades, says, however, that Kligman was a "fascinating person" with "two speeds—bloody genius or wrong."[46] Dr. Rudolph Baer, another aging titan of the profession and former chair of New York University's dermatology department says, although he has never worked intimately with him, he has known Kligman "all [his] professional life" and has heard colleagues refer to him as everything from a "scoundrel to a genius."[47]

His students were enormously impressed with him; Dr. Kligman departed from the dry, austere demeanor of research professors. "He was a maverick," says Dr. Isaac Willis, a resident at the University of Pennsylvania medical school in the late 1960s.[48] "He was different. If anybody would do things it was Kligman. He was brilliant and very good at motivating an individual and challenging me." Dr. Paul Gross, a University of Pennsylvania medical student in the late 1950s, also considers Kligman a "genius" and "one of the few" in the field "who is really creative and original."[49] He believes Kligman should have his own "foundation to discover new ideas and ways of doing things."

But Gross and others were also aware of a troubling side of Dr. Kligman. "He told students that rules don't apply to genius. They just get in the way of creative minds," says Dr. Gross. "He thought he could do and say anything and get away with it [because] he was superior to the average fellow and deserved greater freedom. As a student, I believed everything he said. Later, I realized that a lot of what he said was self-serving and ridiculous." Dr. Gross was not alone in his perceptions. "I was a big Kligman fan," says Dr. A. Bernard Ackerman, perhaps the pre-eminent dermatopathologist in the country, of his early infatuation as a newly arrived second-year resident with the noted dermatologist; his admiration for Kligman was the reason he had chosen to do training at the University of Pennsylvania.[50] "He was famous and had a lot of style and pizzazz, but another resident warned me that the fascination would wear off. It did and I completed my residency at Harvard after spending only one year at Penn."

Part of the Kligman "pizzazz" was a personality and physical constitution that matched his scholarly abilities. According to those who knew him, he had enthusiasm and an electric-like intensity; he was a bundle of energy and in superb physical condition. An outstanding gymnast during his college days at Pennsylvania State University, it was said he could still walk on his hands at age 50. In a 1988 magazine article, the writer described Kligman as "an effervescent man who seems to radiate energy, bombastic opinions, and good humor."[51] "At 71 he looks at least 10 years younger. His skin is tanned from time spent on the tennis court." Even those who have known him more intimately over an extended period of time consider him a natural "showman and entertainer."[52]

The manner in which he would arrive for his inspections of Holmesburg's medical experimentation unit would draw intrigued looks and hushed tones. Alan Katz says, "Kligman had a little scooter and would visit the prisons on it."[53] Alex Gougnin says he saw the doctor enter the institution "in his riding britches" and high leather boots as if he had just hitched his horse outside the prison wall, and, occasionally, the doctor would "fly a plane and land at the Northeast Philadelphia Airport" before making his regular inspection rounds at the prison.[54] And former Holmesburg inmate-photographer Al Butler claims he saw Kligman arrive at the prison in a helicopter. "Helicopters were a novelty at the time and you could not help but notice someone arriving in one."[55] Dr. Kligman's arrival at formal gatherings was also guaranteed to attract attention. Calvin Triol recounts seeing him give a lecture to a "prestigious society in a bathing suit. He'd leave a swimming pool and come right to the lecture in his bathing attire."[56]

During Dr. Kligman's early years at Holmesburg, his experiments were fairly rudimentary dermatological studies, but a growing portion of his work concerned topical applications of experimental creams, oils, lotions, deodorants, detergents, shampoos, and other potential commercial products that pharmaceutical firms hoped to market. And prisoners were well on their way to becoming the lab animals of choice for the burgeoning drug industry. As one observer who has monitored drug company machinations over many years asserts, "Prisoners were used because they were cheap and nobody gave a damn what happened to them."[57]

V

Access to the inexpensive prison population was critical to the industry's scheme for product development. Food and Drug Administration (FDA) regulations dictated that all new drugs pass through a series of experimental hurdles to determine their effectiveness and potential side effects. The three-stage testing process began only after the proposed drug had successfully completed a series of animal tests. In the first and riskiest Phase I stage, the new compound called the IND (investigational new drug) is tested on a small group of healthy individuals to determine the drug's effect on the body's metabolism. If no toxic properties are discovered and the drug still appears promising, it passes on to Phase II, in which a more substantial group of normal subjects are tested with gradually increasing dosages until the limit of safety has been determined. In Phase III, the new drug is given to a larger number of subjects, usually patients, in order to test its efficacy as a disease fighter and to assess its market potential.

Prison inmates had become such an integral part of the preliminary testing that they constituted nearly 100 percent of the Phase I experimental populations across the country, according to Dr. Alan B. Lisook, former chief of clinical investigations for the FDA.[58] Physicians with prison practices or connections to a prison were in demand and could look forward to substantial income. Dr. Milton Cahn shared the Holmesburg site with Dr. Kligman. Drs. Cahn and Kligman were neither strangers nor cut-throat competitors; they had a student-teacher relationship for a number of years. Dr. Cahn explained in a recent interview that he had been in general practice after World War II, but decided to take on a specialty and go back to school in 1951 when he was 33 years old. He says, "Penn was the elite place to go...the most prestigious" and had a program "set up for guys coming out of the Army....We were older, more mature, out of the service with a background in internal medicine...and Penn was the esteemed program in the nation."[59] As a chief resident between 1952 and 1954, Cahn had the opportunity to take a mycology course with Kligman and calls it "one of the best organized lectures [he] ever received."

While a resident in dermatology at Penn, a member of the faculty, Dr. Walter Shelley, asked Cahn if he would be willing to "assist him at the prison" with a series of studies that Shelley was conducting. Shelley's offer was Cahn's introduction to prison research and led to an offer from "Pfizer in New York to run tests" for them. Reflecting on the events four decades later, Cahn calls his clinical research in prisons "serendipitous"; the pharmaceutical firms felt Holmesburg would be "an ideal place to do blood studies." They weren't interested in "testing toxicity, just blood levels" for various drugs. Within a short period of time he had so many offers that he started his own firm, the Research Testing Association.

Dr. Cahn says that, at first, he had "a little piece of H Block" at Holmesburg for his studies, but eventually moved his research operation to "A Block at the House of Correction for isolation" purposes. He describes his program as a "tight, very professional operation" that employed "eight or nine people to watch all facets of the program." He emphasizes the safety of his research: "[There was] never a toxic factor involved in [my] studies. I didn't want to get involved in Phase I studies. We just did Phase II blood studies. We were highly ethical and aboveboard."[60]

By the late 1950s, Cahn's research program had become a partnership when he was joined by his brother Dr. Burt Cahn, a psychiatrist by training. In a recent interview, Dr. Burt Cahn says, "I started independent of my brother, but later became partners with him."[61] The pharmaceutical houses "Hoffman-Larouche, Parke-Davis, Abbott, Lederle, Pfizer, and Smith, Kline & French...contacted me [and] hired me" to run clinical experiments at Holmesburg. He says he tested "a host of anti-anxiety medications and tranquilizers...Librium, Valium, Atavan, Lerax, Haldol, and a variety of sleeping pills" on the prisoners.

Dr. Burt Cahn worked at Holmesburg from 1959 to 1965. He gives two reasons for his departure. The first involved a "career choice: stay as a psycho-pharmacologist" or become the practicing psychiatrist that had been his original intention. "I chose the latter," he says. The second issue was his personal safety: "I became concerned about the growth of the Muslim movement." The Nation of Islam, or Black Muslims, as they were more popularly called, grew dramatically in the 1960s as America's prisons became an arena for recruitment and training in black nationalist and racial separatist ideology. Under the passionate and often confrontational leadership of Elijah Muhammad and Malcolm X, Muslims learned an antiwhite philosophy and a paramilitary code of behavior that many white prison employees found threatening. "Islam in the prison," a force with which he no longer wished to contend, combined with a "very taxing and time consuming" work schedule that had him doing "all [his] own research...even on Saturdays and Sundays," and Dr. Cahn decided to leave Holmesburg Prison.

His brother, Milton, on the other hand, faced a possible ouster because of his proximity to Kligman during the FDA's investigation of Dr. Kligman's research. In July 1966, the high volume of Dr. Kligman's research program had triggered an FDA investigation into his data and record keeping. Although Cahn's program was completely separate, and much smaller, he was caught in the preliminary investigation.

Dr. Cahn says he was brought to a special meeting at Holmesburg that included Kligman, the warden, and the FDA investigators. "They quizzed us for over an hour. I kept denying we had anything to do with Kligman's program, but they wouldn't believe us. They confiscated all my records and examined them. We suffered the pangs of doubt for over a year," says Dr. Cahn.[62] But what was especially frustrating for him was Kligman's silence. The respected doctor refused to tell the FDA that Dr. Cahn did, indeed, operate a completely separate research program. "Kligman never said a word," recalls Cahn. "It was terrible."

Cahn said his research program was put on hold until finally, "after a year, [the FDA] said we had done nothing wrong...[and] were cleared." Though exonerated, the experience forced Cahn to acknowledge the potential professional risk of his proximity to Kligman's high-profile and more diversified research enterprise. "We abandoned Holmesburg," says Cahn, matter-of-factly. "I knew we had to find our own penal institutions for scientific studies." Nearby prisons in Bucks and Lancaster Counties became the new sites for Cahn's Research Testing Association.

Despite this painful episode, Cahn still credits Kligman for "unilaterally [raising] dermatology to its high status today....Dermatology was in the basement, [there was] no respect. We were called pimple squeezers. They made jokes about us: 'How long does it take to learn dermatology?'...'Three weeks.'" Kligman, he says, admiringly, changed all that. He "brought in students from all over the world...and elevated the science of dermatology."[63]

VI

Throughout the 1960s, Albert Kligman's empire in clinical experimentation was growing rapidly: he procured more commercial and governmental contracts, initiated more experiments, recruited more inmates as test subjects, and hired more medical personnel to manage the operation's busy schedule. The program had even captured the attention of the media that described to Cold War America, always responsive to displays of patriotic fervor, the novelty of convicted criminals sacrificing their well-being to science. One newspaper article from 1963 began: "When American soldiers—and civilians—are better protected from the effects of chemical warfare it will be thanks to a University of Pennsylvania doctor and several dozen inmate volunteers at Holmesburg Prison."[64] The article goes on to describe experiments designed to study how "poisonous vapors" penetrate the skin, a study involving "radioactive isotopes [and] a special [climate] cell." The newspaper accounts from the early 1960s were positive, upbeat articles that praised the program and extolled the virtues of prisoners who volunteered to wear "strips of adhesive on arms, legs, and backs, or have small plastic cups bandaged to their skin [so that researchers could study] baldness...aging skin...[and] allergic reactions to various drugs such as the 'mycins.'"[65] All of the articles pointed out as well that the inmates "get paid for what they do." As the author of one article stated plainly, "It would be a mistake to report that most offer their services altruistically...they can earn anywhere from $20 to $500 a year."[66]

There was no threat of having to depend upon inmate altruism; each year brought additional contracts, more products to be tested, and more money. In 1959, the inmates earned a total of "$73,253 by volunteering to take pills, get poison ivy and use creams and salves."[67] Most of these inmates were still earning standard wages for standard tests—"a blood study might mean $5 or $10, a biopsy $5"—but some were now participating in more unusual experiments. Just two years later, in 1961, the total inmate income more than doubled as "prisoners were paid $166,000 by Penn for acting as guinea pigs in various tests."[68] One hundred inmates volunteered for a 1961 Army study, funded by a $21,000 research grant to the University of Pennsylvania Medical School, to measure "the effects of heat and humidity on the human skin." The prison system allowed the university and the Army to build "a special climate chamber...in one of the prison cells" where the temperature could be "raised to that of an African jungle or lowered to almost zero."[69]

Kligman's wife at the time, Dr. Beatrice Troyan, directed one of his few female experiments. Contracted to measure the "maximum absorbency" of sanitary napkins, Dr. Troyan, an obstetrician gynecologist, was brought in to "freeze and weigh" discarded pads for the local paper company.[70] According to Dr. Kligman's FDA file, one problem-ridden contract that used his wife's medical skills resulted in his becoming "considerably embarrassed" and suffering "real distress" from an unsuccessful experiment begun in the summer of 1963.[71] The private-sector sponsor thought it "convenient" to have Dr. Troyan perform their "proposed evaluation" on a compound that had already received "human and animal" trials.[72] Designed to determine "the tolerance of the human vaginal to daily insertions of medicated and unmedicated suppositories,"[73] the test subjects would consist of "one hundred healthy adult institutionalized females"[74] from the women's unit at the House of Correction. By October,1963, however, the study had taken a wrong turn and was being described by the contractor as an "unfortunate miscarriage of the protocol" due to "the misunderstanding of the experimental methods and the dosage regimen by Dr. Troyan and the personnel at the Philadelphia House of Correction."[75] Although the study's sponsor considered this error "regrettable," they hoped to "salvage some information regarding the acute toxicity and pharmacologic effects" of the experiment by asking Dr. Kligman to collect as much data as possible about the "incident." Kligman admitted "responsibility" saying, "we made a serious error" on the "first thirty-three patients," and informed the sponsor that "no charge will be made for this portion of the study."[76]

Correspondence between Dr. Kligman and the sponsor throughout the rest of the year concerned Kligman's inability to supply the sponsor with the data and documentation the sponsor thought necessary, as well as items they believed were required for the FDA.[77] One request referred to the need for individual "patient release forms"[78] and Kligman wrote back: "Our inmates sign release forms devised by ourselves. I cannot make them available to you. This a restriction imposed upon us by the civil authorities. We are particularly hampered in dealing with female inmates. Our projects are carried out as quietly as possible."[79] By late december 1963, the sponsor was still requesting information about the experiment and its impact on the test subjects. Apparently disconcerted by the endless stream of requests, Kligman replied: "I tried to make clear to you that the case records were kept as composite notes on the entire group and are not in a form which I feel prepared to submit for inspection. You also know that I am considerably embarrased concerning some of the errors and imperfections of this study."[80] He went on to claim that "while there is much to criticize, the dominant findings...that this agent cannot be considered for marketing...are trustworthy and real." Kligman concluded his letter by pleading: "You can continue to embarrass me by requiring individual case records which we do not have in a presentable form (and which I do not know for certain are not obligatory to the FDA), and by pointing out the unhappy events which have characterized this project from the start: Yet, I am hopeful that we can count on your understanding and sympathy."

Five days later, the sponsor fired back a less than sympathetic response.

> Please allow me to clarify my position. I have not at any previous time been informed by you or Dr. Troyan that individual case records were not kept in this study. You will recall that our Protocol specifically requires the maintenance and submission of individual case reports. Our desire to obtain these reports does not relate alone to FDA reporting requirements but to our own desire to obtain the maximum information regarding the expected findings of [name undisclosed in FDA copies of correspondence].
>
> You must recognize that our concern with your objective findings is scientific and not dictated by marketing considerations. We do not reject your observations but simply seek to clarify the events resulting in unexpected [undisclosed].
>
> It is the consensus of our Research Department that this study deviated from the protocol agreement in so many important respects that not only should no further payments be made, but that a refund of the advance, in so far as it exceeds out-of-pocket expenses, should be requested.[81]

Dr. Kligman wrote back:

> I deeply regret having irreversibly alienated you. Nonetheless, I am truly shocked by your suggestion that [you] be relieved of paying the cost of this study...we put much time and effort into this study [which was] far from worthless....Our costs were substantial and your unwillingness to be even slightly sympathetic appears to be exceedingly cruel....My own proposal is that you should pay fifty percent (50%) of the original estimate...the information you received is worth at least this much.[82]

Despite occasionally strained relationships, the Holmesburg Prison medical research program grew in scope and sophistication with each passing year, so that by the mid-1960s the research unit not only had the climate chamber—referred to by the inmates as a "space ship"—but also the capability to study numerous radioactive isotopes, conduct unprecedented dioxin testing, and administer sophisticated experiments for the Army. While the more mundane tests such as deodorants, detergents, hair dyes, diet drinks, and the like were still the backbone of the operation, Kligman had now broadened his research enterprise to include a number of more unusual and risky medical adventures.

Many of these new experimental initiatives had nothing to do with Dr. Kligman's specialty of dermatology. In the mid-1960s, for example, R. J. Reynolds Tobacco Company began research into the metabolism of tryptophan and drew volunteers from the company as well as nine inmate volunteers hired by Dr. Kligman. According to R. J. Reynolds:

> RJR initiated research seeking to verify an hypothesis advanced by a Canadian researcher, Dr. W. K. Kerr, that the reported statistical relationship between smoking and bladder cancer could be explained because smoking may alter the body's normal metabolism of tryptophan—one of the eight essential amino acids. Specifically, Kerr and his associates speculated that smoking might lead to increased concentrations of compounds called ortho-aminophenols, which were thought to be associated with bladder cancer. The RJR studies —conducted with both animals and humans—addressed only the fundamental biochemical hypothesis whether smoking led to an increase in ortho-aminophenols in urine.
>
> The RJR research group was faced not only with developing research methods to explore this hypothesis, but also with identifying animal models that would mimic human biochemistry. Further since the hypothesis could only be confirmed with human studies, it also included volunteer smokers. Some of the volunteers were company employees. A Philadelphia research laboratory managed the nine non-employee volunteers, who were local prison inmates. Diets of both the animals and volunteers were supplemented with tryptophan to increase the researchers' ability to measure its metabolites in urine samples, which were taken during periods of smoking and nonsmoking.[83]

The "Philadelphia research laboratory" used by RJR was Ivy Research, a private firm founded by Kligman in the early 1960s. Fortunately for the prisoners, according to Reynolds spokespersons, "in the end, neither the animal studies nor the human studies confirmed the underlying biochemistry of the Kerr hypothesis, and the project ended."[84]

VII

Dr. Kligman was very busy. In 1966, his associate and protege Dr. Chris Papa presented a paper at the annual meeting of the American Society of Dermatology in Chicago that praised the results of a new topical treatment for hair growth using testosterone. The oral presentation at the dermatological society was an outgrowth of a *JAMA* article that had appeared early the previous year. Entitled "Stimulation of Hair Growth by Topical Application of Androgens," the article co-authored by Papa and Kligman described "an indisputable demonstration of at least partial regrowth of hair" on the heads of the "residents of the Riverview Home for the Aged" (of which Dr. Papa had become the medical director) "and the inmates of the Philadelphia County Prison."[85] *JAMA* editors were so alarmed by this "modest investigative report" that they cautioned their readers in an editorial:

> Until more exhaustive clinical experience is obtained, the potent capabilites of testosterone, which is one of the few substances well absorbed through intact skin, should deter most physicians from adding the cream to their armamentaria. Salt and water retention, virilization of women and their in utero female offspring, other endocrine imbalances, testicular atrophy, prostatic hypertrophy, and stimulation of androgen dependent prostatic carcinoma, all possible consequence of such therapy, consitute dangerous reefs in these uncharted waters.[86]

Many years later, Dr. Kligman would defend himself by arguing: "The prisoners insisted that it grew hair, and I was taken in by their enthusiasm."[87]

Although such incidents were no doubt embarrassing, and pointed to his occasionally lax methodology, Kligman combatted theoretical setbacks with a full-court academic press: he churned out so many articles on so many topics that the less credible studies were lost in the mountainous verbiage of all the others. Some of his papers—of which there are many hundreds—could be lengthy affairs on rather mundane subjects such as the dynamics of hair loss[88] or the impact of phototoxic drugs on humans,[89] while others resembled quick commercial advertisements that hardly warranted publication. An example of the latter was his two-paragraph piece on the attributes of the Johnson & Johnson Band-Aid. Based on his experience in "thousands of patch tests," the plastic Band-Aid had proven "wonderfully convenient and useful."[90] In a classic Madison Avenue pitch, Kligman informed his colleagues: "Band-Aids are simply and quickly applied, best of all they stick to the skin tenaciously even in the face of sweating or showering." Moreover, the Johnson & Johnson product was "superior to its rival" from Curity because "the square of the former [is] backed by a cottony material, while the latter has only some additional folds of gauze." Other publications were on topics considerably less onerous to the test subjects than many other experimental ventures taking place inside the institution. For instance, one study dealt with the impact of chocolate on acne. In this experiment, 35 inmates were given chocolate bars for a month to determine if that substance "aggravates acne." To the delight of the Chocolate Manufacturers Association of the USA, who sponsored the study, Kligman concluded "the ingestion of high amounts of chocolate did not materially affect the course of acne."[91]

It was because of studies such as these that many critics believed Kligman's Holmesburg research to be superficial and flimsy, certainly not serious science. Alexander Capron, a former law professor at the University of Pennsylvania and the first executive director of the National Commission for the Protection of Human Subjects of Biomedical and Behavioral Research, which was established in 1974 in the aftermath of congressional hearings on human experimentation, had the impression the Holmesburg inmates were "treated like white rabbits" in order to gauge their "reaction to drugs" of interest to the pharmaceutical industry.[92] Unaware of Kligman's work for the Army, he believed Kligman's prison experiments were "cloaked in medical research and science, but really trivial" in their impact on scientific knowledge. In his estimation, "the prisoners were really used as guinea pigs" and the experiments they volunteered for "did not really ennoble them" as had the prison studies designed to combat malaria during World War II and polio and cancer in the postwar period. The Holmesburg inmates, he believed, were recruited not so much "for science, but for commercial reasons. The inmates were being exploited for pay."

VIII

Of course, poor methodology can be just as dangerous in trivial as in important studies. One example that was of critical importance to the research program and actually threatened its existence was the previously mentioned Food and Drug Administration investigation of Kligman's testing procedures in the mid-1960s. At its heart, the issue concerned what Calvin Triol referred to as Dr.

Kligman's tendency to "start a test and cut it prematurely" if preliminary results supported his hypothesis.[93] This was the crux of the physician's dilemma when the *Philadelphia Sunday Bulletin* printed a mid-summer, 1966 story saying that "Holmesburg prison's world-famous medical research facility is in doubt" and all further drug tests were banned.[94] The FDA specifically charged Dr. Kligman with "failure to comply with the conditions applicable to the use of investigative drugs, in that records and reports of drug investigations have been found to contain irregularities."[95] The reading public learned from the *Bulletin* article of four points that concerned the federal agency:

1. A 26-week study ended after 16 weeks, and the number of subjects involved was less than what was reported.

2. A test subject who withdrew from the study because of a "severe adverse reaction" to the test drug was not reported.

3. Questionable blood studies were supposedly drawn from inmates who were not in the prison hospital when the samples were taken.

4. There were no records for a study that was reported.

Much of the controversy centered on DMSO (dimethyl sulfoxide), which had recently come under greater scrutiny and was banned from human testing by the FDA. A by-product of the timber industry, DMSO had become a universal solvent, facilitating the absorption of other drugs into a person's blood stream. According to Dr. Alan B. Lisook, the investigator for the FDA, "[DMSO] could be rubbed on one's skin and in a very short time would be smelled on the person's breath."[96]

Dr. Frances O. Kelsey, the FDA's chief of the IND branch of the division of new drugs, says "DMSO was being used in veterinary medicine" and in humans for a multitude of physical ailments ranging from everyday "aches and pains" to "painful bladder conditions." She said the drug created some "interesting psychological effects" and was so "widely abused" that it eventually "triggered congressional hearings."[97]

Dr. Kelsey, who is credited with preventing thalidomide from being marketed in the United States (it later proved to cause major birth defects if taken by pregnant women) reportedly was curious about the high number of studies Dr. Kligman was initiating at Holmesburg and "wondered how accurate work could be under such mass production conditions?"[98] Kelsey's curiosity was unsurprising. Between 1962 and 1966, the Holmesburg research program had conducted 193 studies. "Used in the studies were 153 experimental drugs, including 26 drugs for which firms were seeking marketing permission and 14 others whose makers wished to market them for new uses."[99]

One of these inmate studies drew the scrutiny of the FDA because of its prominent appearance in the Fall 1965 issue of the *Journal of the American Medical Association.*[100] The two-part, 15-page article on the controversial chemical DMSO (used as an anti-inflammatory and topical analgesic) was like a red flag to FDA investigators. That really "did him in," recalled Dr. Lisook.[101]

On July 19, 1966, the FDA notified 33 drug firms sponsoring Holmesburg experiments that Dr. Albert Kligman no longer was acceptable for drug testing. The firms included some of the largest in the Philadelphia area such as Wyeth Laboratories; Merck, Sharp and Dohme; and Smith, Kline & French Laboratories. They were told to call back any of their samples still in Kligman's possession. In their notification, the FDA said:

> We have information which leads us to conclude that Albert M. Kligman, M.D., President and Director of Clover Labs, Inc., Ivy Research Labs., Inc., and Betro Labs., Inc., Philadelphia, Pennsylvania, has failed to comply with the conditions applicable to the use of investigational drugs....
>
> You are notified that Dr. Kligman and all investigators associated with the three named corporations are not eligible to receive investigational new drugs.
>
> You should recall any investigational new drugs you may have shipped to Dr. Kligman or the named corporations.[102]

By the end of the month, 75 percent of Holmesburg's test projects had been abruptly dropped and the program administrator in the prison, Solomon McBride, said: "If we don't get relief from somewhere soon, we'll just dry up."[103] McBride was not alone in his expression of dismay. "This is a valuable program from our standpoint," said Superintendent Hendrick. "I would hate to lose this."[104]

The superintendent's concern was modest compared to those in the pharmaceutical industry who were dependent upon the inexpensive prison testing program for large, unfettered, human drug studies. "This facility was badly needed by us," said one spokesman for a large drug firm. Another referred to it as "irreplaceable" and feared that the site had been destroyed by the FDA's action.[105] No one interviewed the test subjects for their reaction at the time, but it was reported that the research operation "placed $115,000 into the pockets of prisoners" during the first six months of 1966;[106] there must have been some regret at its loss.

According to numerous physicians who were University of Pennsylvania dermatology residents at the time, Kligman went into a severe depression and was not seen at the university or the prison for lengthy periods of time. The FDA sanction, and its embarrassing publicity, signified a crippling blow to the doctor's reputation and career. *Time* magazine, for example, devoted a full column to Kligman's research debacle, underscoring that "for only the second time in its history the Food and Drug Administration [has] struck a physician's name from its approved list of researchers who are entitled to test new, investigational drugs on human subjects."[107]

Based on similar FDA rulings, Dr. Kligman's prospects for continuing his lucrative prison research program appeared slim. The *Philadelphia Bulletin* reported an FDA spokesperson's response to a question about the success of an appeal: "Since Dr. Kligman already has made a direct appeal to the FDA...it doesn't look as though he's very likely to succeed in another try."[108] As if by divine intervention, however, the FDA restored Dr. Kligman's privileges to investigate new drugs less than a month after their initial action against him. Letters signed by Winston B. Rankin, deputy commissioner of the FDA, were sent to the 33 drug firms advising them that the restrictions placed on Dr. Kligman's work by the FDA on July 19, 1966, had been lifted. The agency advised the drug companies that "since [July 19] Dr. Kligman and his associates have instituted a number of significant changes in their procedures which makes it possible for us to now regard Dr. Kligman, and the investigators associated with the three named corporations eligible to receive investigational-use drugs for clinical testing."[109]

Dr. Kligman's ability to rapidly rise from his research grave was not lost on FDA investigators. "It was unique to be reinstated at that speed," says Dr. Frances Kelsey when asked about the incident.[110] Her colleague, Dr. Alan Lisook, is equally impressed: "It was very unusual to be reinstated that quickly."[111] He calls it a "singular case"; it was, in fact, the "only case" he can recall where someone was "disqualified and reinstated in that short a time." When questioned about the reason behind Dr. Kligman's quick reinstatement, he identifies "the pressure brought to bear" by significant members of the medical community, namely Drs. Donald M. Pillsbury and Luther L. Terry. Dr. Pillsbury was one of the great names in the field of dermatology, an emeritus professor, and a highly respected former chairman of the department at the University of Pennsylvania; Dr. Terry was the vice president of medical affairs at the university, but more importantly, was the former U.S. surgeon general.

Though the FDA's Lisook was under the impression that Luther Terry was the key architect of Kligman's reinstatement, others in the Philadelphia area gave the credit to Donald Pillsbury. Solomon McBride says, "Pillsbury went down and got to the FDA. He was a big, powerful man" and was able to reinstate the testing program.[112] Kligman's "got a big mouth. He got us in trouble." McBride remembers Dr. Kligman making "some demeaning remarks about" Dr. Frances Kelsey and further admits, "I don't think anybody was supposed to work with [DMSO]."

Regardless of who engineered Kligman's reinstatement, part of the agreement with the FDA, evidently, was an act of penance in the form of a public apology for his lax scientific reporting. On September 26, 1966, *JAMA* published a letter from Dr. Kligman in which he admitted a "regrettable inaccuracy" in his DMSO research, "owing to inadequate supervision on my part," and stated that the test results were "not fully supported by the experimental procedures."[113] Kligman admitted that the test in question—a 24-week study during which DMSO was applied each day to the entire trunks, from chin to pelvis, of 20 inmates—actually ended at 16 weeks, with some men slipping out earlier and one man experiencing "giant hives on the trunk at night" that was not reported. Undeterred by his admission of sloppy scientific methodology,

Kligman tried to maintain the original thrust of his study, and "the sum of accumulating experience seems likely to sustain the conclusion of low topical toxicity." The FDA, however, did not share the doctor's opinion that DMSO was safe enough for further experimentation with humans. Their official position remained that the risks are greater than the potential benefits, and the FDA halted testing in humans.

In a 1992 interview Kligman talked about the FDA ban: According to Kligman, an inmate at the prison where the research was conducted exaggerated the number of subjects in the study without Kligman's knowledge. "I became the victim of a scam."[114]

After Kligman was reinstated, the Holmesburg experimentation unit went back to full capacity almost immediately, which pleased inmates, prison officials, Kligman's medical staff, and, of course, the pharmaceutical companies. Dr. Lisook says there were only "minor problems after that, nothing major," thereby allowing Dr. Kligman to return to his high volume drug studies.[115] In fact, Lisook recalls, "Kligman may have done more testing than any other doctor" in the country. "If he wasn't number one, he was up there."

IX

In retrospect, the 1966 FDA/Kligman imbroglio was a watershed in the dermatologist's lengthy and productive career. A stern, irrevocable sanction by the federal agency might have harnessed, if not curtailed, some of the experimental abuses that were to follow. Similarly, greater care and oversight by the University of Pennsylvania might have prevented what would result in a series of embarrassing revelations years later. To better understand the operations of the FDA and the University of Pennsylvania at that time, it is instructive to look more closely at the FDA sanction of Kligman and his reinstatement.

According to FDA files, the Kligman investigation arose in the fall of 1965, when a discussion of "suspect clinical investigators" was to be held before the Drug Research Board of the National Academy of Sciences.[116] Of the six investigators under examination, records showed that Dr. Kligman "was studying the highest number of investigational new drugs" and was performing "work from a total of 33 different companies....The stimulus to investigate Dr. Kligman" gained momentum after it was reported that "severe hematologic changes" had occurred during "clinical trials with one topical preparation. The inability "to get a satisfactory response" to inquiries about these trials led to an inspection of the site.

Internal FDA documents show that their investigators found numerous scientific and methodological "irregularities," including:

1. "Irregularities or falsification of reports in at least four studies."

2. "Dr. Kligman, a dermatologist, has been involved in a number of investigations involving fields other than in his specialty."

3. "The practice of using an inmate to participate in more than one drug study at a time e.g., a dermatological and an internal drug at the same time."

4. "Serious discrepancies in the record keeping."

5. "Kligman has been involved in a very large number of investigations [experiments]."[117]

As the investigation progressed, several meetings were held between Dr. Kligman and FDA investigators. At one meeting where the shortcomings of the DMSO experiment were being examined, Kligman is reported to have surprised his inquisitors by admitting: "If you think this study is bad, you should see some of our earlier ones."[118] An FDA memorandum dated May 19, 1966, reveals the following exchanges in another conference:

> He [Kligman] stated that the studies were originally done chiefly with inmate help, but now outside civilian personnel were used instead. He said the business of drug testing had grown "logarithmically." He said he realized we had found one or two errors in testing, but he thought in general his work was reliable. Dr. Kelsey pointed out to him a number of serious discrepancies....Dr. Kelsey expressed our concern over the toxicity findings in a recent [undisclosed] skin product which were not reported promptly and [from which] the blood slides...were destroyed. Dr. Kligman felt this was a breakdown in communications only, since the man in charge of this study was used to studying only "inert" compounds such as soaps....Dr. Anderson pointed out that a number

of subjects in drug testing also were used in extensive skin testing and expressed doubt that possible adverse effects could be separated out.

Dr. Kligman acknowledged these errors but felt all his work couldn't be condemned. He said "we could ruin him" but he didn't see how we would want to do it on the basis of so "few mistakes." He said he thought the least reliable of all his studies were the dermatologic ones since these, until recently, were not done under the medical adminstrator, but under his own supervision. Dr. Kelsey expressed shock at this since she said we all felt his reputation was chiefly in the field of dermatology....

Dr. Kelsey felt that she had to (and nothing in the meeting had changed her mind) recommend to the Commissioner that Dr. Kligman was not an acceptable investigator until he brought evidence that the situation in his testing set-up was such as to inspire our confidence.[119]

On July 22, 1966, three days after Kligman had been declared "ineligible to receive [new] investigational drugs," Kligman and his attorney met with the FDA leadership to protest the "harsh sentence."[120] Various excuses were offered for his noncompliance with regulations governing new drug studies, including faulty record keeping by inexperienced personnel, depending too greatly on "prisoner help," and poor supervision, but the sanction remained.

According to FDA files, Kligman's chief defender and the individual most responsible for his reinstatement was Dr. Donald Pillsbury, who informed the FDA that the "results of this sudden declaration of ineligibility of Dr. Kligman have been absolutely catastrophic."[121] Pillsbury claimed the action "has been a coup de grace to [Kligman's] personal, professional, and financial standing, and has necessitated the sudden dismissal of several very worthy people." In addition, he argued, "it has removed a highly effective morale-builder at Holmesburg Prison." Pillsbury described his colleague as "a very imaginative and productive clinical...investigator [with a] worldwide reputation." Pillsbury was "convinced that Dr. Kligman has not been guilty of any misrepresentation," and that any "errors" that were made were "inadvertent." He concluded by saying the closure of the Holmesburg research laboratory would be a terrible loss: "There are relatively few competent facilities capable of carrying out tests on volunteers."

On August 4, 1966, high-ranking FDA officials visited Holmesburg in order to hear Dr. Kligman and Dr. Herbert Copelan (the medical director of the research program) present "a series of proposals" prepared in the hope that they would "tighten up" the program and bring it into compliance with the FDA regulations for INDs.[122] The 14-point plan discussed a cross-section of issues covering record keeping, the volume of work, supervision, consent forms, and oversight committees. The FDA officials were unimpressed: many of these proposals were supposedly in place when the investigation began and "really constituted no change in the organization."

Later that day, however, the FDA investigators "paid a courtesy call" on Dr. Luther Terry, the former surgeon general who was now the vice president of the University of Pennsylvania for medical affairs.[123] Dr. Terry told the investigators his "chief interest" in the Kligman case was "in preserving the good name of the University of Pennsylvania." He said he had learned from Dr. Isadore Ravdin, his predecessor at the university, as well as others that, "while Kligman was eager and an entrepreneur, that he was thought to be fundamentally honest." However, Ravdin did relate to Terry his "great concern" that Kligman was "trading upon the name and reputation of the University of Pennsylvania in his private dealings with drug firms and others concerned with his drug testing program." The FDA investigators thought this of "some interest" since those who investigated the Holmesburg research program had noted that "all the prisoners employed in Dr. Kligman's research unit—which does commercial testing—wear a uniform which is clearly labeled 'University of Pennsylvania Research Unit.'" Dr. Terry concluded his meeting with the FDA officials by telling them that the FDA action had placed him on "a very warm if not actually 'hot seat'" and he hoped it would be resolved as soon as possible.

In fact, it was. Just over a week later, Dr. Pillsbury was volunteering his services as an "unprejudiced advisor" in order to bolster Kligman's 14 proposals and regain FDA compliance.[124] In a rapid series of phone calls and written correspondence, Pillsbury pledged to "review all protocols...final reports, and make spot checks at the prison facilities." Pillsbury wrote, "My willingness to undertake this task is based on a strong conviction that Dr. Kligman and his associates have a basically sound and valuable investigative facility. I am willing to expend considerable time and effort to restore it to operation, and to aid in making it as impeccably accurate and reliable as possible."

Three days later, on August 15, 1966, an internal FDA memorandum stated: "It appears that the newly initiated procedures are adequate to satisfy our requirements."[125] Dr. Kligman had escaped a career-threatening blow; the obstacles had been overcome. A handwritten note by W. B. Rankin, the acting commissioner of the FDA, on his copy of the memorandum, reported that he had notified Dr. Pillsbury of the change, and Dr. Kligman was once again eligible to receive investigational drugs. Dr. Pillsbury, it is noted, said he "would help keep close watch over the clinical trials that are carried out."

In the subsequent months, Rankin received a series of "This is just to let you know" letters from Dr. Pillsbury, informing him how the new procedures were working at the prison. Pillsbury related that he "found everything in good order"[126] and "came away with the feeling that the studies are going ahead very well indeed."[127]

Kligman had received a new lease on his life as a scientific researcher. Though somewhat battered by the experience, his reputation slightly tarnished by his clash with the FDA, he was able to resume investigating new drugs for pharmaceutical companies and explore hundreds of new protocols using thousands of prisoners.

X

Despite the controversy that surrounds him, there are many who speak with warmth, reverence, and appreciation of Dr. Kligman and their Holmesburg experience. Calvin Triol was hired by Kligman and the University of Pennsylvania after he had dropped out of Hahnemann Medical School in Philadelphia. He had hoped to stay in the medical research arena, and after a short stint at Wyeth Labs was sent to the University of Pennsylvania by an employment agency and became an integral part of the human experimentation program at Holmesburg. Hired in 1964, Triol claims to be the third employee recruited by Kligman outside of his medical school retinue. He believes Kligman's initial years at the prison centered on purely academic interests, but as the years passed, the testing took on a life of its own, attracting major corporate clients and requiring additional staff and test subjects. Triol ran tests for Kligman at both Holmesburg and the House of Correction, and by the time he left the program in 1969, he estimates 30 civilians were employed as experimentation support staff.

Triol refers to Kligman as his "mentor" and his Holmesburg tenure as "the springboard to the rest of my career" in clinical experimentation.[128] He remembers "working 80 hours a week and [loving] it"; he calls the whole experience "tremendously stimulating and exciting." Triol says, "[the research program] was...totally positive, for us, the inmates and the institution....We were all young and in a growing, exciting situation." He firmly believes the human experimentation program was a valuable asset, especially to the inmates. "Without the testing program the prisoners had nothing. It improved life within the prison." With pay from participating in the tests, the inmates "sent money to their family, bought toiletries, and hired attorneys."

Triol emphasizes that payment to the inmates "was only a portion" of inmate benefits from the research program. He lists a host of other enhancements: "it allowed inmates to get off the block"; it improved the function of the prison; it alleviated "the boredom that leads to riots"; and it gave the inmates a sense of being "helpful" and "contributing to research." Of course, he admits, some "inmates tried to use the testing program for their own purposes"; inmate recruiters acquired power and payoffs. Finally, he argues, until the testing program, the prison health care operation was "incompetent, uncaring, and underfunded....The inmates benefited from the testing program because it brought in solid support staff" and modern, state-of-the-art medical equipment.

As for the experiments themselves, Triol believes they were harmless and contributed to advancing medical science. For the most part, he said, they were "household products such as toothpaste, deodorants, detergents, and so on." Kligman decided which tests the prisons would agree to do, and each warden gave final approval. Ed Lyons, a superintendent of the city prison system in the late 1970s, and a veteran of the system over four decades, disputes this: "Wardens did not give approval of a protocol."[129] The only aspect of the experiments that wardens controlled was "the movement of the inmates and the location of testing."

Triol was the head of the satellite testing program at the House of Correction where Lyons was the warden in the late 1960s. Triol firmly states that "the warden had to sign-off and Lyons refused on a couple of occasions....We would summarize the full protocol in layman's terms so the warden could understand [the experiment] and if the warden said no, [or had some objection to the test,] "Kligman would say, 'don't worry, we'll do it at Holmesburg.'"[130]

Triol says he sometimes advised the warden against running a test. "He and I would agree on what tests were safe." When he occasionally found a test "distasteful," he chose not to do it. Triol also confirms that there were isolated instances when people were "kept in the dark about the tests," but cautions that contractual obligations "bound [the researchers] to remain silent."

Calvin Triol claims that the times when prisoners were placed in hazardous conditions were rare. He also says he was unaware that dioxin experiments were taking place in the prison, but if so, he argues, Dr. Kligman was the "ideal person in the world" to perform the tests. "He was the place to go," says Triol, proudly boasting of his mentor's status. He is less enthusiastic about the Army studies, about which he claims to know little and is reticent to discuss. His hesitance centered on testing that went far "beyond Dr. Kligman's area of expertise." Kligman, Triol says, "was not qualified" in mind control and experimental psychotropic agents.

Alan Katz was the pharmacist for the medical research program at Holmesburg for eleven years until it closed in 1974. Katz attributes his career in clinical testing to his father-in-law, who was the lay Jewish chaplain at the city jail. Aware of the burgeoning testing program, the chaplain told his son-in-law, who had just received his degree, about an opportunity in the prison system. Katz "interviewed two or three times at Penn's Duhring Labs" on the college's West Philadelphia campus and was hired shortly thereafter.[131] When he started in 1963, Katz noticed that "inmates were dispensing medication" to other inmates. Katz says, "It didn't strike me as smart." The authorities had a higher level of confidence than he did that the inmates would actually swallow the pills rather than market them back on the cell block.

He says "that policy changed in time and more civilians were hired" to handle tasks that prisoners had been performing.

Always present in large numbers, apparently, were the future dermatologists of the world, medical students and hospital residents who trained under Dr. Kligman's direction at Holmesburg. According to Katz, there was a strong "international" flavor to the Penn medical staff, with many "European, South American, and Asian" doctors working in the program.

All in all, Katz says, the program "did a lot of good things for thousands of people." And the testing back in the 1960s was ethical. The inmates had a choice. "They didn't have to participate. They could say yes or no." In addition, their participation was a "wonderful source of income" that provided "spending money" for an assortment of commissary items that made life inside the jail a little more hospitable. He admits that the inmates received "slave wages" from the program, but argues that the pay was still considerably more than the prisoners were earning at regular institutional jobs.

Katz laments, "It's a different ballgame today....The Helsinki Guidelines and a half-dozen other guidelines today" have changed the business. "Informed consent has evolved over the years and a band-aid study today would require a 7-page informed consent declaration."

Alan Katz claims he didn't know they were giving psychotropic drugs to the inmates involved in the U.S. Army experiments. "I wasn't involved in that program," he assures me. "It was somewhat secret." He claims he specifically kept his distance from the trailer experiments because of their quasi-secret status and their negative reputation around the prison.

Solomon McBride was Dr. Kligman's right-hand man and managed the testing program on a daily basis for its two-decades-long existence. McBride began his career in penal work in the early 1950s dispensing drugs (though he lacked pharmacology certification) but found his true career niche a few years later when Dr. Kligman hired him to help establish and administer the research testing program in the prison. He was viewed as "a very competent guy" and an able administrator.[132] McBride says, "Some of my finest hours were spent in Holmesburg. We helped a lot of people in that program." He claims "nobody was injured in those tests." They were all "non-invasive procedures." "We never broke the skin on any of them." He points out proudly that "we were sued and we never lost a court case." McBride repeatedly stresses the innocuous nature of the tests, offering studies on "Crest toothpaste and Coast soap" as examples. When asked specifically about more dangerous experiments, he either denies that they were conducted or denies knowledge of them. Holmesburg prisoners, for example, took part in dioxin and mind-altering drug experiments. "Even I wasn't aware of that," said McBride. "I don't believe it. I don't think it ever happened." When asked about the use of radioactive isotopes, he is quick to respond. "No that wasn't done. I don't think the prison would permit it." Informed that documents from the Atomic Energy Commission verify the use of isotopes in Holmesburg,[133] he admits, "I heard about it, but I don't know anything about it."[134] McBride emphasizes that he was "not aware of everything that went on there," and launches into a declaration of his concern for the well-being of the inmates. "I was opposed to things that were not kosher. If I saw something wrong, I'd tell 'em to stop. I told the residents [doctors] not to do stuff that was dangerous." Referring to the medical staff, McBride says "If they hurt those black brothers...I wouldn't let them do it."

Outside of Kligman, the most important of the many doctors associated with the institution was Herbert W. Copelan. Dr. Copelan, the research program's medical director, was a no-nonsense physician who is said to have run a tight ship. Whereas Dr. Kligman traveled up to the Northeast Philadelphia site of Holmesburg to visit his experimental ventures once or twice a week, Copelan and McBride were at the prison on a daily basis and actually supervised all aspects of the busy and diverse research program. Alan Katz says, "Dr. Copelan's day-to-day procedures were rigid" and he was meticulous in his conduct of the experiments contracted by Kligman.[135] In Dr. Katz's view, Copelan is a consummate professional and extremely competent. "He was terrific," very deliberate and confident in his approach, Katz says admiringly. "Many of the inmates could not meet the standards" for participation in the experiments because of drug use or other disqualifiers. Copelan "would reject 25 prisoners to get one good candidate," Katz recalls.

Katz and Triol agree that while most of the research staff had limited knowledge of the exact experiments, Dr. Copelan must have been one of the select few to have considerable knowledge of the substances prisoners were being given. The controversial Army tests, for example, that Katz and Triol claim to have little knowledge of, was an area Copelan had direct medical control over. Unfortunately, Dr. Copelan refuses to discuss his experiences at Holmesburg, and says news articles and public interpretations have distorted his actions and resulted in painful allegations.

XI

With the forced closure of the Holmesburg medical experimentation program in 1974, research staffers were aware that prisons as clinical test sites were no longer viable. The 1970s and 1980s ushered in tougher federal restrictions on human experimentation and past practices were widely criticized. Although much of the criticism came from politicians, lawyers, and bioethicists, they have now been joined by medical colleagues who worked in the penal institutions alongside the experimenters, but in more conventional healing capacities.

"It's shocking and abominable," states Dr. Mel Heller, when told the full story of testing at Holmesburg.[136] "It is next to impossible to get informed consent from individuals in a dependent state. Prison inmates are very vulnerable." A prison psychiatrist for several decades, Dr. Heller started many of the first penal psychiatric programs in the Philadelphia area and worked at Holmesburg during Dr. Kligmans's long tenure there. Dr. Heller says of Kligman, "He was making big bucks and a small amount was going to the prison." "It was dreadful, [basically selling] flesh for a sum of money. Prison inmates should not be used in medical experimentation unless very unusual protections [can be offered]." Heller says the "pound of flesh syndrome" is "entrepreneurial" and develops in an atmosphere in which "extremely aggressive pharmaceutical and medical industries form phenomenal alliances, similar to the military-industrial complex." Heller emphasizes that "those were the days when they didn't care about the inmates....A research project has to be benign and have the inmates' interest at heart....If you don't, you could do grave harm." He says that in a system that offers few ways to make money, the uneducated, vulnerable inmates with histories of risky behavior "would gravitate to the medical tests and actually compete for a part of Kligman's operation." When asked why so few individuals attempted to caution the inmates about the tests or why knowledgeable observors in the medical profession kept silent about the risks involved in the Holmesburg experiments, Dr. Heller could only reply: "Who knew what they were doing?"

Dr. Heller's knowledge of the medical research program, however, was broader than most of the staff's. In 1967, he authored a comprehensive, detailed article on the subject for *The Prison Journal*, a publication of the Pennsylvania Prison Society, of which he was a board member. Entitled "Problems and Prospects in the Use of Prison Inmates for Medical Experiments," the article addressed such issues as informed consent, free choice and free will, the element of risk, financial rewards, and several other key aspects of the increasingly controversial practice.[137] The prison psychiatrist cited some of the medical experiments that were underway in the prison system. They included:

1. "A number of tranquilizers, analgesics, and antibiotics" that were being tested for "dosage and toxicity" for various pharmaceutical companies.

2. A "dental study" for Johnson & Johnson that included "one hundred inmates" testing toothpaste and mouthwashes for "toxicity." Inmates received "twenty to twenty-five dollars, plus two dollars extra for any blood tests."

3. A "wound healing study" for Johnson & Johnson in which the "absorbency and wound-adhesion properties of various dressings" were examined. Inmates were "paid five dollars per wound."

4. An "antiseptic lotion study" for Johnson & Johnson that utilized seventy inmates.

5. An antiperspirant preparation for Helena Rubenstein that paid twenty inmates at the House of Correction two dollars per day.

6. A "napkin absorbency study" for DuPont that paid 150 female prisoners 50 cents for each used napkin that was frozen, saved, and returned to DuPont.

7. Numerous skin "sensitization" studies including a "sodium lauryl sulfate" solution that left inmates with "broken skin, swelling...and pustules." The test subjects received thirteen dollars for twenty-eight days of participation.

Dr. Heller also developed a sophisticated list of conclusions and recommendations about the "medical-experimental program," including the observation that the prison system was owed $45,388 that the research program had paid the city for the use of its prisoners. That figure was a percentage computed from "approximately $272,329 paid out to prisoners for their participation in medical experiments in the fiscal year of 1966."

In conclusion, Dr. Heller's article argued for a more meaningful relationship between experimenters and test subjects. "As active partners, sharing equitably in the frustration and rewards of research, there is more good than money that can come from such a program."

Dr. Arthur Boxer, also a psychiatrist, has spent four decades working with inmates in Holmesburg and other area prisons. He was quietly mystified by the human experimentation program. "I was always concerned about it, but I wasn't a whistle blower. I was fairly new at the game at the time."[138] He says he had "no idea what they were testing," but for the inmates, it was "better than the usual way to make money," which translated into "14 cents an hour."

Dr. Boxer says he was impressed by the level of "craziness" going on around Kligman's experimentation program and believes that such an operation "could never, ever happen today." Interestingly, Boxer is not automatically opposed to prisoner experimentation, even though he claims to be aware of tremendous "inequities," "bribery," and other "rumors" about the Holmesburg experiments. "If it is a well-designed program and there is informed consent and reasonable understanding, I've no problem with it," he says. But Boxer underscores the need for informed consent in prison "like you'd give informed consent anywhere else. You have to respect who you're dealing with, even inmates."

Another psychiatrist with many years of experience in the Philadelphia prison system is Dr. Edward Guy. He too speaks of "ambivalent feelings" about the former experimentation unit.[139]

Kligman "was very helpful...very sophisticated. Any problem you had, they'd take care of." But Guy also "heard rumors" about the trailers and "Department of Defense" work that used "mind-altering drugs, hallucinogens," and other potent chemicals. Dr. Guy admits that prisoners were good "research candidates," but you "can't take a guy without a lot of free choices. Research today is totally different from back then."

The psychiatrists recognized the entrepreneurial underpinnings of Kligman's experimentation program. "I knew he was making a pile of dough," says Boxer, who calls the research program a "fabulous plum" and a "major source of good things" through its revenue potential. "He's a sharp animal," Boxer says of Kligman's ability to develop medicine into a lucrative business.

The financial enticements of such business arrangements can be considerable. Dr. Aron Start, a professor of medicine at the University of Wisconsin and the former medical director of the Texas prison system, asks: "Do you know how seductive some of this can become to work for government and money?"[140] Start, who has served as an expert witness in numerous court suits concerning prison medical standards, says that clinical research is "well defined now," but it had a "sordid history in this country" because of a "distorted view of those individuals who are incarcerated." He says "prisoners were viewed as appropriate subjects" because they were perceived as "less valuable." It was "clearly unethical behavior."

Al Bronstein, director of the ACLU's National Prison Project, goes considerably beyond Dr. Start's criticism, comparing domestic prison research programs to the experimental studies orchestrated in "Nazi Germany."[141] He says actions such as Dr. Kligman's at Holmesburg were "outrageous, unethical, and morally indefensible....You can't get voluntary consent from inmates. It's the same as the doctors at Auschwitz." Unfortunately, he says, doctors like Kligman were all too common in America after the war. The public felt if famous doctors like Albert Sabin could perform experiments on prisoners, then "it must be valuable" and all right.

Calvin Triol, on the other hand, looks back fondly on his years with Kligman and believes he was doing a "patriotic service that was good for the public and the country."[142] Solomon McBride asserts: "I've got a clear conscience. I've got nothing to hide."[143] And Dr. Albert Kligman remains unshaken as well.

From Kligman's point of view, the Holmesburg research program was good for both medical science and the Philadelphia prison system, "quite beneficial to all."[144] He includes the inmates as beneficiaries of the research. He believes that without the testing, inmates' lives would have been devoid of the human relationships and outside stimulation that the research program provided. "People said the inmates weren't free to make a choice....It was said that the prisoners were coerced by money," but that wasn't true, argues Kligman.[145] And when it is mentioned that the inmate volunteers were paid well, especially by prison standards, Kligman quickly agrees that indeed they were. "The money was an important inducement to the inmates. Inmates went out [of prison] with hundreds of dollars," but the program gave them "much more than a source of income." Kligman emphasizes that it was "a welcome addition to prison routine," which is boring and repetitive and lacks any professional or cultural stimulation. We brought in people they could talk to, says the doctor, meaning his medical staff. The program fostered "greater social activities"; it was an "antidote to boredom." Kligman talks about the skills that the inmates learned and that enabled them to get jobs on the outside when they were released. Kligman claims he helped many of them do just that. An additional contribution was a "well-stocked pharmacy" that carried the latest medications for a population that normally would not have received such state-of-the-art attention.

All of this, according to Dr. Kligman, was good for prison management. The prison did not benefit financially. "What they got back," he says, "was a better run, more manageable prison." As Kligman views it, the sad demise of the program was "a very good case of the triumph of the do-gooders." The do-gooders are those "liberals, lawyers," prison reformers, and opponents who made his experiments into "a Nazi-like thing....All we did...is offer them money for a little piece of their skin." But the experiments got "a bad name" and became "a dirty word." Kligman says he was hurt and outraged that he had to listen to people call him a neo-Nazi. "I'm Jewish! It struck me as ludicrous and incredible that I'd be compared to that."

In *Kind and Usual Punishment*, Jessica Mitford's 1973 landmark study of American prisons, a sobering look at prison inmates as human guinea pigs was presented to the American public for the first time.[146] Her revealing account informed readers that the scientific establishment in the United States had never totally embraced the Nuremberg Code and many imprisoned citizens were being abused in the name of medical science. In my discussions with her, she repeatedly drew the analogy between prison researchers in America and the Nazi physicians placed on trial after the war.[147]

For two decades—from the early 1950s to the early 1970s—Philadelphia's Holmesburg Prison played host to one of the largest and most varied medical experimentation centers in the country. Only the inmates, and the doctors who experimented on them, know just exactly what took place, but whereas the latter choose not to discuss their earlier medical exploits, the prisoners are not asked. In that respect, Holmesburg is little different from the dozens of other institutions that contained vulnerable populations and were exploited in the name of scientific advancement. This sad but widespread twentieth-century phenomenon has much to teach us about our ethical standards and our capacity for human compassion.

Part Two

TWENTIETH-CENTURY AMERICAN PENAL EXPERIMENTATION

Three

"They're Dropping Like Flies Out Here."

I

On August 20, 1947, Gerhard Rose, one of Germany's pre-eminent medical figures, stood in the prisoners' dock at the Palace of Justice in Nuremberg, Germany, awaiting his sentence for "murders, tortures, and other atrocities committed in the name of medical science."[1] The prestigious German physician had overseen a series of experiments at the Buchenwald and Natzweiler concentration camps, in which numerous healthy inmates were deliberately infected with yellow fever, smallpox, typhus, cholera, and diphtheria germs. Hundreds of these inmates died.

Gerhard Rose was one of 23 defendants at the Doctors Trial, which began on December 9, 1946. More than eight months of graphic testimony revealed a broad range of "ghastly" and "hideous" high-altitude, malaria, mustard gas, bone transplantation, sea water, sterilization, and incendiary bomb experiments. The men accused of using "numberless unfortunate victims...as human resources for nefarious and murderous purposes" represented the elite of German medicine. Siegfried Handloser was chief of the medical services of the Armed Forces. Paul Rostock was chief surgeon of the Berlin Surgical Clinic. Karl Brandt was the head of S.S. Medical Services and Adolf Hitler's personal physician.[2] The other 20 defendants had reached similar positions of authority and prominence; they were now accused of murder and were on trial for their lives.

Dr. Rose, who was the department head for tropical medicine of the Robert Koch Institute, "became exasperated" during one phase of the trial when the chief prosecution witness, Dr. Andrew C. Ivy of the medical school of the University of Illinois, continued to reiterate the basic principle "that human experimental subjects must be volunteers."[3] In reply, Dr. Rose vehemently argued that the United States was guilty of similar practices and enumerated several examples in support of his provocative contention. His knowledge of American medical history may have saved his neck: he escaped the hangman's noose and was given a life sentence.

II

The Nazi doctor's first illustration of America's own experiments with prisoners occurred in the Philippines, then an American Territory, in the early years of this century. In 1906, Dr. Richard P. Strong, an American who was the director of the Biological Laboratory of the Philippine Bureau of Science, performed a series of experiments with the cholera virus upon the inmates of the Bilibid prison in Manila. The experiments resulted in 13 deaths. A government report attempting to explain the embarrassing affair said Dr. Strong had "made some remarkable discoveries with reference to cholera serum" and had "used it with success on various occasions," but that in administering it to some 24 inmates of the penitentiary of Bilibid, a bottle of "plague serum was probably substituted for a bottle of cholera serum."[4] It is believed that Strong, who later became professor of tropical medicine at Harvard, "obtained the permission of the Governor of the Philippines, but not of the victims, to infect with plague a group of criminals condemned to death."[5] The doctor was "thoroughly convinced" that man could withstand the same amount of plague organism as a guinea pig and argued that the "human inoculations were performed as carefully and with as much deliberation as possible."[6]

Although he was initially distraught over the disastrous incident, Dr. Strong, a graduate of Yale and Johns Hopkins Medical School, used prison inmates six years later to perform experiments with beriberi, "a deficiency disease characterized by paralysis, mental disturbance and heart failure."[7] These experiments, too, resulted in several deaths. The survivors were rewarded with cigars and cigarettes.

Of course, not all medical experiments were conducted quietly offshore. To learn whether sulfuric acid, which is used in making molasses, might be injurious, the Louisiana State Board of Health put "Negro prisoners on a steady diet of molasses for five weeks."[8] Few in the community thought this practice alarming. One account stated that, the inmates didn't "object to submitting themselves to the test, because it would not do any good if they did."

Indeed, some members of America's university and scientific community were vocally and publicly offended by the cavalier behavior of doctors toward prison inmates. But a writer in 1907 responded to criticism with the following: "The most curious misconception [is] that the aim of science is for the cure of disease—the saving of human life. Quite the contrary, the aim of science is the advancement of human knowledge at any sacrifice of human life."[9]

A Navy doctor who stood alongside Gerhard Rose in the prisoners' dock at Nuremberg was Georg August Weltz, an accomplished physician and chief of the Institute for Aviation Medicine in Munich. Dr. Weltz was on trial for his "special responsibility for and participation" in high-altitude and freezing experiments at Dachau.[10] Weltz—who was acquitted and freed—mentioned in his defense the experiments of Dr. Joseph Goldberger, a U. S. public health official, who sought to unravel the mystery of pellagra. In 1914, the state of Mississippi recorded almost 1,200 deaths from pellagra, a disfiguring, deadly disease that was particularly virulent in the deep South. The following year, more than 16,000 reported cases resulted in over 1,500 deaths. Those unfortunate enough to contract the disease often suffered the four "Ds": dermatitis, diarrhea, dementia, and death. Complaints of "listlessness, weak knees, pain in the back and neck, a burning sensation in the stomach and extremities, and an inflamed and sore tongue" led to reddening of both hands and feet and an ugly skin rash across the face—pellagra's distinctive signature.[11] Conventional medical wisdom at the time blamed everything from poor sanitation and personal habits to spoiled corn and flawed hereditary traits for the disease. With little real insight into the origin of the "red flame" or its treatment, victims of pellagra were outcasts, shunned in most places and treated little better than lepers during the Middle Ages.

Impressed by Goldberger's innovative approach in other areas, Governor Earl Brewer of Mississippi "authorized a new pellagra experiment" using inmates in the state prison system. The research would be carried out at Rankin Prison Farm, eight miles east of Jackson, Mississippi. Dr. Goldberger's plan was naively simple: "induce pellagra in white adult males, the one group in the population that statistics had shown was the least likely to contract the disease." The doctor believed that a good diet prevented pellagra and a bad one induced it, but he needed to prove it. He was convinced that the South's regional diet, especially for the poor, of fatback (meat), meal, and molasses supplied calories but not necessary protein. Milk, vegetables, and fresh meat, Goldberger theorized, were the missing staples. It was not a starvation diet that was killing so many southerners, but the lack of a nutritious one. The dozen Rankin Farm inmates who volunteered for the test, after the promise of a governor's pardon, became his experimental guinea pigs.[12]

The "pellagra squad" was organized in February 1915 and consisted of "six who were serving life terms for murder, one a life term for criminal assault, and the others lesser terms for manslaughter, bigamy, and embezzlement." The dozen volunteers were sequestered from the other inmates, but did the same work: cutting weeds and grass, sawing lumber, and painting buildings. Their diet, however, differed considerably, and by late summer the men had grown sick from a steady diet of corn bread, mush, collards, sweet potatoes, grits, and rice. Complaints grew as most of the men suffered from pains in their backs, sides, and legs, and from increased lethargy and dizziness. Many of the men begged to be freed of the experiment and returned to the general prison population, but Goldberger would not allow it. They had volunteered; they would have to stay the course regardless of the physical consequences. By mid-September the first skin lesions began to appear and by the end of the month all of the men showed signs of a rash on their hands, faces, and scrotums, the typical markings of pellagra.

Governor Brewer kept his word and pardoned the men at a formal ceremony. One relieved volunteer said, "I have been through a thousand hells" and added that he often would have welcomed a bullet in order to be done with the test. Others said they would have welcomed a "lifetime of hard labor" rather than go through such "a hellish experiment" again. Upon their release, the men were offered free medical care until they fully recovered; tellingly, they rejected the offer to see more doctors and "went off like a lot of scared rabbits." The governor received some criticism for permitting the test, although state residents were less concerned about dietary supplements than they were that the convicts had been set free. An untroubled Dr. Goldberger asserted that "science and humanity were forever in [the governor's] debt."[13]

The accused Nazi physicians revealed other examples of human experimentation in the United States: nontherapeutic medical initiatives using prisoners. Most had been carried out no more secretly than Goldberger's pellagra experiments, which concluded with a public ceremony. In California, hundreds of prisoners were taking part in bizarre testicular transplants between 1919 and 1922. These experiments were designed by Dr. L.L. Stanley to test if lost potency of aged and ill men could be reinvigorated. Five hundred of San Quentin's inmates had testicular transplants, some with "animal glands" of rams, goats, and boars surgically implanted in their scrotum. Dr. Stanley said it was "fortunate that this work could be carried out in a prison, for in such a place all men are treated alike, and live under the same conditions of food, work and general surroundings."[14] There is little record of what the test subjects thought of the experiments, but on their behalf Dr. Stanley, who promised "to pursue the truth, wherever it may lead," argued that the procedure promoted general "bodily well-being" and was "practically painless and harmless."[15]

In another case, twelve years later in 1934, the nation learned the story of Carl Erickson and Mike Schmidt, two Colorado prisoners who were selected to participate in unprecedented tuberculosis studies at Denver's National Jewish Hospital. Though fearful of the drug trials, Schmidt said, "I don't exactly relish the idea of making an experiment of myself."[16] The men managed to survive the experiment and Governor Edwin C. Johnson rewarded them with a pardon. However, Johnson's pardon was criticized by some; one citizen wrote, "we fail to see any excuse for releasing upon the community two life-term fellows because they didn't get tuberculosis when inoculated with a preparation of microscope bugs."[17] Four years later, *Life* magazine covered the story of a condemned Utah prisoner who allowed physicians to record the duration of his heart function after being shot through the heart by a firing squad.[18] Clearly, although a blind spot for American observers, sufficient precedents for human experiments had been set by American doctors to warrant the connections made by the Nazi doctors.

III

For the most part, the use of inmates for medical experiments was still rare during the 1920s and 1930s, still medical oddities generally devoid of both research ethics and public concern. But the uncommon practice received a significant boost at the outbreak of World War II. With American soldiers fighting and dying in Europe and the South Pacific, a whole new industry utilizing human resources was about to emerge that would profoundly affect researchers' behavior for decades to come. The experimental endeavors would be considerably larger—broadscale clinical investigations that were adequately funded and well-staffed. Just months before Pearl Harbor, President Franklin Roosevelt created the Committee on Medical Research to discover antidotes for such diseases as influenza, malaria, and dysentery—diseases devastating the troops. Over the next four years, the government would appropriate some $25 million that would swell the coffers of hospitals, colleges, and corporate institutions. The establishment of research sites capable of testing dozens of volunteers at once became a significant hurdle. For the nascent medical-pharmaceutical industry, the appeal of penal institutions became overwhelming. By appealing to their patriotism, prisoners were solicited for the necessary human trials testing remedies to diseases like malaria and typhus, and techniques in skin grafts and exotic blood tests. Some of these medical initiatives were bizarre and the results tragic. In the summer of 1942, for example, the U.S. Navy, with support from Dr. Edward J. Cohn, a distinguished Harvard biochemist, made a pitch for volunteers at a state prison in Norfolk, Massachusetts. The prisoners were told that the war had created a blood shortage of plasma and volunteers were desperately needed to test a substitute derived from beef blood. The test involved injecting each volunteer with an ounce of purified fraction of beef blood. Nearly a third of the institution's 750 inmates volunteered, the vast majority of whom had fewer than two years to serve until parole. Sixty-four men were injected, before the experiment was stopped. Twenty of the men became ill from serum sickness, eight seriously, "with high fever, rashes, and joint pains. One was dead."[19]

In New York, scores of Sing Sing Prison inmates volunteered for daily doses of unfamiliar drugs, like atabrine, to help the Army determine whether, under the drug's influence, soldiers could carry full workloads.[20] New Jersey supplied the Army with enough willing prisoners to host a series of experiments including sleeping sickness, sand-fly fever, and dengue fever.[21]

Probably the best-known example of human experimentation in a state prison—and one prominently mentioned by the Nazi physicians on trial at Nuremberg—was the case of Stateville Penitentiary in Illinois. Beginning in September 1944, when Dr. Alf S. Alving of the medical school of the University of Chicago, first asked if "inmates of Stateville might be willing to volunteer as experimental subjects...in an effort to find a cure for malaria," more than 400 prisoners participated in the intensive, two-year-long study.[22]

While many articles describing the experiments were published in such journals as *The Journal of Infectious Diseases*, one of the best layman's accounts of the Stateville malaria experiments are the two chapters in Nathan Leopold's book *Life Plus 99 Years*. Written by one of the infamous convicted killers in the 1924 Leopold and Leob case, the book delivers a step-by-step account of the research program's origin and development, as well as the "dangerously sick" fevers the inmate volunteers had to endure. Leopold emphasizes the patriotic and altruistic motivations of the test participants and the unique collegiality of the keepers and the kept. "Not the least remarkable feature of the project," he writes, "was the fact that it put the administration and the cons on the same side of the fence, partners in a common endeavor." He was certain "that many volunteers derived more solid, lasting satisfaction from what they were doing than many of them had known in some time."

The inmates had to contend with periodic mosquito bites, raging fevers, nausea, vomiting, blackouts, endless untested medicinal potions, and occasional relapses, but "no one squawked. They all took it like men." A team of *Life* magazine photographers went to the prison to capture the human drama for the general public, whose attitude was not to ask if the men had given their free and informed consent, but to congratulate these patriotic lawbreakers.[23] As one newspaper proudly put it, "these one-time enemies to society appreciate to the fullest extent just how completely this is everybody's war."[24]

As was becoming more common, test subjects signed informed consent or waiver forms that allowed authorities to claim participants understood what they were getting into and absolved the authorities of any untoward results and legal repercussions. The Stateville malaria waiver stated:

> I...hereby declare that I have read and clearly understood the above notice, as testified by my signature hereon, and I hereby apply to the University of Chicago, which is at present engaged on malarial research at the orders of the Government, for participation in the investigations of the life-cycle of the malarial parasite. I hereby accept all risks connected with the experiment and on behalf of my heirs and my personal and legal representatives I hereby absolve from such liability the University of Chicago and all the technicians and assistants taking part in the above mentioned investigations. I similarly absolve the Government of the State of Illinois, the Director of the Department of Public Security of the State of Illinois, the warden of the State Penitentiary at Joliet-Stateville and all employees of the above institutions and Departments, from all responsibility, as well as from all claims and proceedings or Equity pleas, for any injury or malady, fatal or otherwise, which may ensue from these experiments.
>
> I hereby certify that this offer is made voluntarily and without compulsion. I have been instructed that if my offer is accepted I shall be entitled to remuneration amounting to [xx] dollars, payable as provided in the above Notice.[25]

At the conclusion of the program, a "considerable" portion of the men received parole, because the governor wanted to reward them for their brave actions. Those with longer sentences and more serious crimes, such as Leopold, "could not be paroled," but the test participants were "all sure that some means would be found to give [them] consideration." Several years after the war had ended, Governor Adlai E. Stevenson granted commutations of sentence or paroles to 317 of the 432 convicts who participated in the malaria tests including 24 murderers and 1 rapist.[26]

Thus it was during the war years that the federal prison system swung into action as a major source of human subjects for research experiments. The U.S. Penitentiary at Atlanta, Georgia, played a critical role in the fight to conquer malaria and approached the challenge as if it were "a major military engagement."[27] The National Research Council, Division of Medical Sciences, and the Committee on Medical Research of the Office of Scientific Research and Development informed the inmates at Atlanta that malaria infection was taking a toll on American soldiers far in excess of Japanese soldiers. And the problem was made all the worse by the enemy's vast territorial holding, which cut off the entire world's supply of quinine, then the best known antimalarial drug.

Approximately 600 of Atlanta's 2,000 inmates volunteered to become "human guinea pigs and undergo malarial infection and treatment with new drugs that were untried on the human system."[28] After a screening process eliminated half the applicants, the rest were "assembled in the auditorium, and informed that every man would become very, very ill, perhaps several times." Although no one was expected to die from the disease, "there was always the possibility of that eventuality occurring in scientific experimentation." Furthermore, as had become standard procedure at this point, the warden emphasized that a convict's participation in the project would in no way "secure or enhance his chance" for an early release.

Men were selected in groups of 15 to be infected by the bites of the anopheles mosquito. Subgroups would be given new preventative drugs prior to the men exposing themselves to at least 10 bites from mosquitoes that were proved infectious. By the experiment's end, 130 men had participated in the project. "One hundred and five were infected with mosquito-induced temperate zone vivax malaria, 15 were inoculated by bites of mosquitoes that had been infected with a New Guinea strain of vivax malaria, and the remaining 10 men given one or more intravenous injections of blood taken from other malaria volunteers during attacks of malaria or during a latent phase of their infection."[29]

Although no one died in the experiment, many of the men probably wished they had, as they contended with a series of relapse and recovery cycles, intensely high fevers, constant aches and pains, and endless blood tests. The volunteers also suffered through eight new medications and the three standard antimalarials—quinine, atabrine, and plasmochon. Nearing the end of the experiment a reporter trumpeted the prison's malaria project as "another shining light in the galaxy of wartime achievements at Atlanta."

Enemies needed to be fought, diseases conquered, and scientific advancement encouraged. Federal prisoners were a rich reserve of human vessels waiting for recruitment in the battle. At Terre Haute, 185 prisoners were enlisted in the fight against gonorrhea, and at El Reno, 300 inmates worked with the National Institutes of Health in "an effort to determine the amount of toxoid necessary to immunize men against the organism that causes gas gangrene."[30] Even juveniles who had run afoul of the law were recruited; the dormitories of the National Training School for Boys were used to test the effectiveness of ultraviolet irradiation of air carrying airborne germs.

Public outcries against these experiments during the war years were few. The overriding goal was to win the war in Europe and Asia; everything else was secondary, including research ethics and the issue of consent. The war became the transforming moment for human experimentation in the United States. Medical experiments on prisoners and other institutionalized groups had been legitimized and there would be no turning back When the war ended, testing in federal prisons subsided but did not stop. The malaria project at Atlanta had ended, but the "National Institute of Health reported highly favorable results," so a similar malaria project was launched at another federal institution in Seagoville, Texas.[31] And by 1949, the Federal Correctional Institution at Danbury, Connecticut, was enlisting prisoners in the fight against infectious mononucleosis, "under the guidance of a U.S. Army medical-research unit working at Yale University."[32]

Medical historian David Rothman has argued that "a utilitarian ethic continued to govern human experimentation—partly because the benefits seemed so much greater than the costs, and partly, too, because there were no groups or individuals prominently opposing such an ethic."[33] Granted, the Nuremberg Code had recently been established, but apparently few were aware of it, and, more often than not, they believed the Code applied only to German doctors. American exceptionalism and our victory in the war worked against any call for a special code of medical ethics—particularly one that presented potential obstacles to America's rapidly emerging scientific dominance. U.S. postwar research wished to be unfettered by a code of medical conduct that proclaimed, as did the Nuremberg Code, the following first principle:

> The voluntary consent of the human subject is absolutely essential. This means that the person involved should have legal capacity to give consent; should be so situated as to be able to exercise free power of choice, without the intervention of any element of force, fraud, deceit, duress, overreaching, or other ulterior form of constraint or coercion; and should have sufficient knowledge and comprehension of the elements of the subject matter involved as to enable him to make an understanding and enlightened decision.[34]

Many interpret this most critical of points to forbid the use of prisoners for medical research purposes; but not a country that had won the war, and whose own medical establishment had not been declared guilty of Nazi-like war crimes. The confluence of self-interest, utilitarianism, and the ideologies of science and medicine militated against the American medical community's immediate embrace of the Nuremberg Code. Prisoners were too valuable as research subjects to be jettisoned. They needed to be used, not protected.

Rothman calls this new era of laissez-faire attitudes in the laboratory "the gilded age of research."[35] Where once the battlefield was the focal point of government concern and resources, medical research would take its place. The eradication of disease had become the new enemy. Postwar budgets supported this goal. In the last year of the war, the National Institutes of Health received approximately $700,000. By 1955, the appropriation had climbed to

$36 million, and in 1970, a staggering $1.5 billion was awarded to some 11,000 grant applicants, nearly a third of which required some form of human experimentation.[36]

If any one individual set the tone for legitmizing human experimentation on prisoners (despite the Nuremberg Code), thereby providing for its rapid growth in the quarter century following the war, it is probably Andrew C. Ivy. An eminent researcher and vice president of the University of Illinois Medical School, Dr. Ivy had been selected as the American Medical Association's official representative and consultant to the U.S. prosecutors at Nuremberg. Medical ethics, as well as general medicine, were said to be his areas of expertise.

On the witness stand at Nuremberg, Dr. Ivy, America's star witness for the prosecution of the doctors, extolled the virtues of human experimentation—at least, as it was practiced in the United States. An earlier witness, Dr. Werner Leibbrant, had argued that imprisoned individuals are, by definition, unable to exercise free will, and cited the Stateville experiments as examples of unethical experiments. Ivy, on the contrary, did not believe that official coercion was necessarily inherent in a prison environment; he maintained that prisoners were offered a legitimate choice between participating, or not, in medical tests. Furthermore, they had the power to exercise that choice. No American prisoner, said Ivy, had ever been used against his will in an experiment.

Nuremberg defense counsel Robert Servatius, hoping to show that American physicians were guilty of practices similar to the medical experiments performed by the Nazi doctors, vigorously pressed Ivy on numerous points, including the wartime use of Stateville inmates for malaria experiments, the coercive effects of offering excessive rewards for volunteering, and the ethics of using inmates sentenced to death as test subjects. In each case, Dr. Ivy defended American medicine; he said "it is not an evil to carry out experiments."[37] In fact, he argued that if practiced as in the United States, medical experimentation is a noble, scientific endeavor and in no way related to the Nazi horrors. In Ivy's view, if "the consent of the subject was obtained," if the experiment was based on "animal experimentation," and if it was directed by "scientifically qualified persons," the medical procedure was acceptable.

Ivy's Nuremberg testimony, and his concurrent efforts on behalf of the Green Committee, which was exploring the medical practices used in Illinois' prisons during the war, considerably muddied the ethical waters. As Ivy had conceded in Nuremberg, prisoners made good subjects because they "had nothing else to do except...render public service....Prisoners in a penitentiary can give their full time...to the experiments, and of course, they are subject to strict control."[38] For American researchers anxious to use the thousands of potential subjects behind bars, Ivy's emphasis on acquiring voluntary consent from participants represented a seal of approval. In fact, such approval was forthcoming less than a year after the Doctors Trial, when the *Journal of the American Medical Association* published a "Special Article" that endorsed the Green Committee's final report and the "ideal" medical practice employed in the Stateville malaria experiments.[39]

IV

It was just four years after the war that *New York Times* readers began to follow the case of a prison inmate who allowed himself to become a human blood-cleaning agent for a young "girl dying of cancer."[40] From a midsummer, front-page story, the public learned of an "unnamed Sing Sing prisoner" who was waiting to see if "he would develop leukemia, one of the most deadly forms of cancer, after having volunteered for a perilous medical experiment" on behalf of a very ill 8-year-old girl. In an effort to "purify the child's blood of the wildly spreading white blood cells characteristic of leukemia," the young girl was brought into Ossining Hospital and laid next to a healthy prisoner. For 24 hours, they lay side-by-side, "their circulatory systems linked together with rubber tubing," and the doctors hoping that the "poisoned blood" in her system would be cleansed as it proceeded through his body. It was estimated that "eighteen quarts of blood" had passed between them. Dr. Charles C. Sweet, chief physician at the prison, said the experiment was conducted to see whether a healthy man's system could absorb cancerous cells without harm to him and on the chance it might save the child's life. Within a few days, the experiment failed—the young girl died. Now the attention shifted to the health of the inmate volunteer. According to Drs. James B. Murphy and Henry Wallenstein of Rockefeller Institute for Medical Research and the Jewish Memorial Hospital respectively, the chances of the unnamed prisoner contracting leukemia were "very, very remote."[41] They both argued that "while leukemia can be transferred to animals," it was less likely in humans. Readers also learned more about the mysterious volunteer: "[he] is 49, reserved, intelligent, and soft-spoken, and has already served fifteen years of his life-term."

In late June, the curious public was given additional information about the brave Sing Sing convict. His name was Louis Boy, and he had originally been sentenced to death on July 9, 1931, for "complicity in the death of a man in a New York hold-up."[42] His execution had been waived by Governor Franklin D. Roosevelt, and his sentence commuted to "life imprisonment." It was further revealed that this was not Boy's first experience as a human guinea pig. During the war, Boy had submitted "to injections of atabrine when its effect in the treatment of malaria was still unknown," and a year later "underwent a test for a new influenza cure." Six months later and just two days before Christmas, Louis Boy appeared in another front-page *New York Times* article: he had just been granted his freedom by Governor Thomas Dewey. The governor said Boy's "exemplary" prison record and his willingness to participate in "dangerous medical tests and experiments...without promise of reward" earned him his commutation.[43] Mr. Boy's service, Dewey said, was "considered an important contribution to the field of medicine." The next day, Christmas Eve, Louis Boy appeared in the paper once again, in a photograph of him leaving Sing Sing Prison. Dressed in a new suit and with satchel in hand, the former lifer, wished all present a Merry Christmas and greeted his 21-year-old son, Joseph. He spoke briefly of his plans and looked forward to choosing one of two jobs he had been offered.[44]

Not everyone was won over by Boy's heroics and the governor's benevolent yuletide spirit. One physician wrote the *Times* a long letter denouncing both the science and the humanitarian gesture behind the much-discussed experiment. Dr. Ludwik Gross, chief of cancer research at the Veterans Administration, wrote that "in the history of medicine [there is] no case on record of a recovery from leukemia. The eventually fatal outcome cannot be prevented. Leukemia, unfortunately, cannot be cured by blood transfusion."[45] Gross went on to criticize the orchestrators of the experiment, arguing that the "risk involved" outweighed any "medical science profit" that may have come of it. He further asked, "was the convict…fully informed that, should the transfusion of leukemic blood result in the transmission of leukemia, his voluntary exposure would be for all practical purposes equivalent to his acceptance of a verdict of death?"

Though Louis Boy was a rarity—an inmate who captured national attention because of his exploits as a human guinea pig—his story was not lost on his fellow prisoners, who hoped for the sympathetic treatment Boy had received. Institutional human experimentation was about to enter its most expansive and unfettered period, a two-decade-long cycle that witnessed numerous medical advances and an equal number of experimental excesses. Human experimentation was about to become "mainstream, legitimate, and a valued activity."[46] The golden age of prison experimentation was dawning.

V

With the arrival of the 1950s and the onset of the Korean War, the federal prison system embarked fully on human experimentation, and numerous penal facilities played host to major research initiatives. In 1953, for example, the following medical projects were underway in the federal system:

1. The malaria testing at Atlanta had "produced highly significant results" and a series of new drugs to fight the disease. More than 400 inmates had been used since 1951 in the "discovery of primaquine and chloroquine as impressive agents" in combating malaria. Early in the Korean war, about 20 percent of returning soldiers had developed malaria after they were back in the United States, but when the new drugs were given to the returnees in a 14-day treatment on board ship, the chances of getting malaria after arrival home were "reduced almost to zero."[47]

2. To combat the high incidence of infectious hepatitis following blood transfusion, the research at Ashland, McNeil Island, and Lewisburg had proved

helpful in understanding that "blood derivative plasma can carry the virus, but that the blood derivatives albumin and gamma globulin apparently do not." This finding "assured...safety in the use of gamma globulin in the...vast drives against poliomyelitis," increased the use of blood albumin, and decreased the use of blood plasma.[48]

3. Prisoners at Leavenworth, Atlanta, and Terre Haute participated in a nation-wide, 20,000-person study for the National Heart Institute to determine the "relationship between the presence of certain chemical constituents in the blood and the development of heart disease."[49]

4. The 175 inmate volunteers at Seagoville, Texas, took part in the experimental transmission of human intestinal protozoan parasites—a study that produced a greater understanding of the transmission of such diseases as amoebic dysentery. The "principal finding" was that "a very small number of eggs of the parasite...can produce infection." This meant that contaminated drinking water is "apparently a far more dangerous source of infection than flies [because] the survival of the parasitic eggs in water was found to last 16 days."[50]

5. Atlanta also worked with the Communicable Disease Center in a large ath-lete's foot study that proved, among other things, that "there is no significant decrease in the incidence of athlete's foot from the use of specially treated shower mats," but "treating shoes with formaldehyde fumes [before] re-issue was an effective procedure."[51]

6. The Federal Reformatory in Chillicothe, Ohio, hosted extensive tests on the common cold. Dr. Victor Haas, head of the Microbiology Institute, said a new vaccine "represented a great surge forward" in the fight against respi-ratory diseases that attack the adenoids, throat, and eyes.[52]

Chillicothe would play an even more prominent and public role in the development of an oral vaccine for polio. Under the direction of Dr. Albert B. Sabin, 133 inmates at the federal Ohio facility had participated in a study of a low-cost vaccine that could be taken by mouth instead of requiring injection. Sabin had been awarded a $1 million grant by the National Foundation for Infantile Paralysis, but it had not given him permission to put on field trials. A new proce-dure using "highly attenuated strains of live polio virus," according to Sabin, was not quite ready for the general public, but would be tested on additional prison volunteers at Chillicothe in late 1956 or early 1957.[53]

VI

State prison systems were not left out of the opportunities for research. Experimentation programs continued as if World War II had never ended, and the number of experiments, test subjects, and prisons involved in medical research grew steadily. And the tests were as diverse as the prison systems.

In New York's Sing Sing Prison, for example, 13 prisoners "donated small pieces of muscle tissue and blood samples for a New York University arthritis study" while another "62 volunteers" spent "fifteen months" being injected with spirochetes of syphilis.[54] In the Illinois State Penitentiary at Stateville, inmates suffered "chills, sweats, pains, and aches" as they endured their own malaria experiment.[55] And Michigan inmates helped Dr. Jonas E. Salk develop a new procedure to rid the influenza virus vaccine of dangerous febrile reactions that were associated with vaccine inoculations.[56]

Female prisoners had their roles. At Clinton Farms, New Jersey's only female prison, 200 women volunteered to participate in an Army study on viral hepatitis. Led by Dr. Joseph Stokes, Jr., of Children's Hospital of Philadelphia and the University of Pennsylvania, the study helped prove that "the virus could be developed in animals."[57] All 200 women contracted the disease after it had been grown in fertilized chicken eggs.

In 1951, the Virginia State Penitentiary in Richmond conducted a series of medical experiments in conjunction with the local medical college to test everything from flash burns, which might result from atomic bomb attacks to, three years later, sophisticated blood tests using radioactive material. The Virginia experiments are interesting for several reasons, not the least of which is the revealing correspondence between the medical school and the prison.

A letter dated October 30, 1951, from Dr. W.J.H. Butterfield to the State Department of Welfare and Institutions, mentioned his appreciation for the valuable service the inmates performed in "metabolic aspects of thermal injury" tests and the recommendation that "you give to each the maximum commutation of sentence."[58] In an earlier letter to the prison superintendent, Dr. Butterfield had explained that "the men will be in the hospital about 20 days, during which time they will receive 16 small shallow burns...to their forearms, and in one instance to their fingertip" from a "strong beam of light in a short space of time."[59]

Prison superintendent W. E. Smyth, obviously sensitive to public disclosure of the experiments at the hospital, wrote Butterfield: "I have informed all the inmates and staff members that no publicity should be given to the experiment being carried on...and the inmates should not have visitors, uncensored mail going in or coming out, and I do not think their name should appear on the daily roster of patients...and by all means they should not have the privilege of the use of the telephone."[60]

The next month the medical college requested two additional "prisoner volunteers" for a blood test that could possibly take "as long as 180 days." Dr. Everett Evans assured the superintendent that "I consider the experiment absolutely safe and have no hesitation in having it carried out on myself."[61] In a subsequent six-page memo on "Observations on Volunteers from Penitentiary," Dr. Butterfield wrote that he faced "these trials [meaning the experiments] with a completely clear conscience," and did not "fear any inquiry," but all the same, advised "the least said the better." Moreover, he suggested placing "more emphasis on the sociological implications rather than experimental implications...to circumnavigate any unpleasantness over these trials."[62]

Doctors and university hospitals recognized their good fortune at the availability of a regular supply of human guinea pigs and did not want a skittish public or curious media interrupting the pipeline. But inmates, too, had a stake in the system. As one prisoner who took part in the radioactive blood test wrote the director of the Surgical Research Laboratory: "I would like to know if a notice, by letter, has been forwarded to the Virginia State Parole Board, in my behalf?"[63] The inmate mentioned that he was "up for consideration for parole [and] under the circumstances, I was very happy to volunteer for the experiments...if volunteers are needed for any further experiments, I will be happy again to be of some use."

Enterprising doctors throughout the country quickly saw the economic potential of such medical-prison relationships. Legal impediments to such ties did not prove insurmountable obstacles. After the Iowa's attorney general ruled that "it was not legal to use prison volunteers" for medical research, doctors in Iowa "sought and obtained...a specific law permitting the use of prisoners for medical research."[64] The law, which passed the Iowa legislature in 1964, allowed men from the Iowa State Penitentiary and the Men's Reformatory to volunteer or withdraw their services at any time. The doctors behind the campaign felt that the "use of prison volunteers for medical research was justified and highly desirable for the investigator, for the subjects, and for society....It not only permits the conduct of human investigation under ideal circumstances, but it enables the participants to feel that they are serving a useful function, as indeed they are."

The Ohio prison system hosted some of the most dangerous and controversial experiments of that period: the injection of live cancer cells into the bodies of prisoners. In coordination with the Sloan-Kettering Institute for Cancer Research and the department of medical research at Ohio State University, inmates volunteered to receive needle injections in the forearm of live cancer cells.[65] This risky experiment was designed to "discover the secret of how healthy human bodies fight the invasion of malignant cells." The researchers did not think the volunteers faced serious danger because the injected cancer cells were not expected to multiply and spread. If they did, "they could be removed quickly by surgery."

Two weeks after being injected with the cancer cells, the infected area of one forearm would be removed surgically for study. The malignant cells remained in the other forearm for an indefinite time. Prison authorities had requested 25 volunteers for this test and 96 responded. Prison authorities called the response a proud tradition. Ohio prisoners had already participated in several other medical studies and, not long before, had supplied 640 square inches of skin to a badly burned little girl who had required extensive skin-grafting surgery.

The live cancer cell experiments in the mid-1950s were under the direction of Dr. Charles A. Doan, director of medical research of the College of Medicine, Ohio State University, and Drs. Chester M. Southam and Alice E. Moore of Manhattan's Sloan-Kettering Institute.

A 1957 *Time* magazine article described each step of the unusual experiment for curious Americans:

> First, Dr. Southam used Novocain to anesthetize an area about three inches across. Into the middle of the area he stuck a tattoo needle that left a blue dot for a reference mark. Out of the vial and into a hypodermic syringe he drew up a cubic centimeter of pink fluid—mostly water, but also containing millions of cancer cells from human victims of the disease. The cells had been grown for years in test tubes by Dr. Alice E. Moore, Sloan-Kettering's tissue-culture specialist....Dr. Southam inserted the point of the needle alongside the tattoo mark and worked it up the arm for an inch and a half, just under the skin. A push of the plunger injected half the syringe's contents (three to five million cells) into the volunteer's arm. Dr. Southam pulled out the needle, turned it around, and repeated the process lower down the arm. (Some volunteers received implants of tissue fragments of other human cancer strains grown in animals and chick embryos.)[66]

Cancer was beginning to receive extensive news coverage as the deadliest disease confronting the American public, and between 1956 and 1958, the *New York Times* printed numerous articles on the bold experiments taking place at the Columbus, Ohio, penal facility. Once again, American prisoners were on the cutting edge of medical science and the general public had become fascinated with their "humanitarian" contributions.

Dr. Southam's cancer cell injection studies would eventually bring him notoriety and a year's probation from the Board of Regents of the State University of New York because of his cancer studies at the Jewish Chronic Disease Hospital. In this well-known 1963 study, Dr. Southam injected foreign, live cancer cells into 22 patients, most of whom were not told about the experiment and many of whom were incompetent to give informed consent. Curiously, the Jewish Chronic Disease Hospital experiments became some of the most notorious and controversial of the era, even though they largely replicated—with the exception of informed consent—similar experiments Southam had undertaken at Ohio State Penitentiary nearly a decade earlier.[67] Once again, prison inmates were a class apart and clearly more expendable.

In a recent interview, Dr. Southam addressed several aspects of his former prison experiments. As with most medical researchers, Southam says that inmates represented a steady, compliant test population. Prisoners, he said, were a "stable group of people" who contributed to the "assurance of continuity" in the scientific process.[68] In his view, it was clearly "more difficult to work with unrestrained, unrestricted" test subjects. But, he says, "prisoners still have rights," and the right of refusal is one of them. The research program adopted "a completely voluntary approach" so no one could argue that he was pressured to become a participant. Southam adds that the "prison weekly newspaper, run by the inmates, [handled] volunteer recruitment." He also emphasizes that the 170 or so inmates who received the cancer injections were unpaid with "no expectation or hope of altering their time of discharge." Southam says: "We did not want people who were coming into it for money. Self-satisfaction was the reward...altruism was the reason they participated. The inmates just wanted to be helpful." Interestingly, when Southam is asked if his prison experiments abided by the Nuremberg Code passed just a decade earlier, he says, "I was unaware of the Nuremberg Code and its code of conduct." Furthermore, "Most of the publicity on the [prison] experiments was favorable during the 1950s."

Not all prison experiments received news coverage. Some remained secret for years, receiving little, if any, publicity. For example it would not be until 1977 that documents revealed that at least 142 inmates at Iona State Hospital in Michigan had been inducted into secret mind-control experiments for the CIA. Apparently, the CIA had given scores of "sexual psychopaths" LSD and marijuana in order "to test the effectiveness of certain medication in causing individuals to release guarded information under interrogation."[69] The U.S. Army and Ohio State University Research Foundation were collaborating on a vaccine to fight tularemia, an infectious disease more commonly referred to as "rabbit fever" or "deer-fly fever." The disease usually causes "an ulcer at the site of involution and enlargement of the lymph glands."[70] Rabbits, squirrels, and other rodents are the usual targets of the disease which is transmitted by the bites of flies, ticks, fleas, and lice. If untreated in humans, death can result, but the test subjects who became ill made a "quick recovery" after prompt treatment with streptomycin. The 31 prisoners in the study received Army certificates of achievement "for risking serious illness to further medical science's fight against infectious disease."

VII

The 1960s brought continued growth in human experimentation in prisons, a rush of new relationships between penal institutions and pharmaceutical companies, and an oversight dilemma for Food and Drug Administration officials. The government itself exacerbated the problem in 1962 when, in the aftermath of the thalidomide disaster, the FDA required pharmaceutical companies to conduct three phases of human trials before allowing a drug to be marketed. Phase I drug testing now required large pools of healthy subjects for nontherapeutic experiments; the former practice of using a few hospital patients was judged totally inadequate. Pharmaceutical companies sought out private or university-affiliated physicians who had access to the stockpile of human material isolated behind high prison walls and living in highly regimented conditions that were rare, if not impossible, to find outside prison walls. A significant bonus for the drug companies and doctors was the fact that the imprisoned masses locked inside these institutions were willing to expose themselves to more risk for less money than the experimental subjects in the outside world. Prisoners tended to be more reckless physically and desperate economically and, therefore, were more willing to accept a fraction of what similar tests paid outside the walls. Finally, government overseers would be less likely to visit fortress-like institutions holding dangerous criminals than tree-lined, ivy-covered college campuses.

Moreover, for those pharmaceutical companies that ran human experiments in the confines of institutions, test subjects getting sick presented far fewer repercussions than did similarly affected individuals on the outside. Most prisoners signed long, complicated waiver forms that placed all responsibility on the test-taker and none on the test-giver. Although such "exculpatory language" would later be declared illegal by various governmental agencies, the legal

subterfuge succeeded in creating an atmosphere of individual pow-
erlessness, a dearth of inmate lawsuits, and greater security and
freedom for the researcher.[71] For Dr. Gerald Wachs, the associate
medical director for Shearing Plough from the mid-1960s to the
early 1980s, the prisons represented a testing site where the subjects were "guaranteed to show up."[72] Wachs says that standard
clinical research in the free world was "worthless if you had somebody for four days of testing and they failed to show up on the
fifth." Clinical experiments at prisons, however, took place in controlled environments that greatly facilitated the testing process. Dr.
Wachs says he could "call up" the prison physician and simply ask:
"Can you do a Draize Test for me? I'd write a check to the doctor
and he'd decide how much the inmates would get."

The relaxed atmosphere coupled with distant governmental regula-
tors translated into an incredible financial opportunity for physicians
with penal practices. One of the most egregious examples of penal
medical abuse is the case of Austin R. Stough, an Oklahoma physician
who farmed the fertile correctional fields of willing test subjects for
several decades. Though Dr. Stough made a fortune—in a good year he
would gross close to $1 million, and the pharmaceutical companies
also profited handsomely—the inmates "sickened and some died in
an extended series of drug tests and blood plasma projects."[73]

Dr. Stough practically cornered the market in the field of prison
experimentation by selling blood plasma extracted from prisoners in
Oklahoma, Arkansas, and Alabama and using the prisoners as subjects for repeated, wide-scale drug tests. It is reported that in the
mid- and late 1960s, he alone oversaw 130 investigational experiments for 37 pharmaceutical companies, including such power-
houses as Bristol-Myers, Merck, Sharp & Dohme, Upjohn, Lederle,
and American Home Products. Some believe him to have conducted between 25 percent and 50 percent of the initial drug tests in the
United States and a quarter of the tests done on a blood process that
created an important plasma by-product used to protect people
exposed to infectious diseases.

Walter Rugaber, a *New York Times* reporter, chronicled Dr. Stough's
odyssey in a lengthy 1969 article that illuminated the doctor's "dan-

gerous methods," the federal government's "indifference," and the pharmaceutical products that could adversely affect "millions of consumers."[74] Dr. Stough began his association with prison medicine in the late 1930s when he opened a practice in McAlester, Oklahoma, site of the state penitentiary. Soon he was serving in a part-time capacity at the prison and "his drug tests began to grow extensively." He added a new wrinkle to his prison practices in early 1962, when he embarked on a plasmapheresis program. The novel procedure not only allowed individuals to contribute blood many more times a year but also enabled plasma to be drawn away from whole blood and the remaining red blood cells to be reinjected back into the donor. The process was a financial windfall for those with access to a large supply of contributors.

The problems were largely for the donor, especially if he fell victim to poorly trained staff and shoddy operations. Tommy Lee Knott, an illiterate criminal, was such a person. Knott's blood type was O-positive, but in a subsequent lawsuit he charged that blood type A-negative had been injected back into his veins after a visit to the plasmapheresis unit. He dropped nearly 60 pounds in 17 days and had liver, lung, brain, and kidney damage, and an assortment of other injuries. Knott sued Dr. Stough for more than a quarter million dollars, but "settled for $2,000 when he went off on a crime spree that landed him in a small town jail."

Only three months later, Dr. Stough expanded his plasmapheresis program into the prison systems of Arkansas and Alabama. Money, illness, and death followed in his wake. The doctor knew how to make friends and business associates of other prison physicians, and was equally adept at co-opting legislative opponents. Dr. Gwyn Atnip was paid $8,000 by the state of Arkansas and an "extra $20,000 a year for his work in the plasma program" by Dr. Stough; state senator Gene Stipe, an ardent opponent of Dr. Stough, underwent a rapid philosophical transformation after being awarded a $1,000-a-month retainer.

By mid-1963, "the incidence of viral hepatitis, an often fatal disease of the liver, was climbing sharply" in the prisons in which Dr. Stough had instituted his plasmapheresis program. As many as 30 inmates a month came down with the disease and several deaths occurred. News of the epidemic began to trickle to the outside world. One inmate said: "They're dropping like flies out here." The doctor and prison officials denied the charges, but the numerical evidence was overpowering. At Kilby Prison in Alabama: "28 percent of the men who participated in Dr. Stough's program came down with the disease. For those who did not take part, the rate was only one percent." The numbers were just as devastating at other institutions used by Dr. Stough.

Federal investigators were less than thorough or vigorous in their investigation, initially following a path of "scientific caution" but ultimately concluding, "Dr. Stough managed a double play: technique and apparatus both were cited in the epidemics."[75]

Pharmaceutical company representatives were less hesitant to state the obvious. One Cutter Laboratory official who visited Dr. Stough's operations said "he was appalled at the situation he found. He said the plasmapheresis rooms were sloppy and that gross contamination of the rooms with donor's plasma was evident." Although Cutter Labs and other pharmaceutical companies had harsh things to say about Dr. Stough's medical operations, none severed their relationship with him. As the Cutter representative said, "Dr. Stough had contacts at the prison and it was through him that permission was obtained from the prison officials to operate the program." Cutter and the other pharmaceutical companies continued to work with Dr. Stough; it would have been too expensive to do anything else. "Oklahoma had taken over the plasma and drug testing programs," but Arkansas allowed Stough three more years of plasma work and never curtailed his drug testing program, which consequently expanded in both drugs and test subjects.

But the tide was turning on Dr. Stough, as more and more questions were asked by government inspectors and newspaper reporters about his businesses. Drug tests were being challenged, procedures questioned, and his qualifications probed. Investigators discovered that some medications like "Indocin, a best-selling product of Merck, Sharp & Dohme, that is used in the treatment of rheumatoid arthritis," was in fact "no more effective than aspirin and produced serious side effects"; dozens of inmates were physically "examined for a new program in just four hours—or, an examination every three minutes"; and testing physicians had "a lot of on the job train-ing...but limited training in basic pharmacology." After an official inquiry, the Alabama Medical Association concluded that Stough's work was "bluntly unacceptable." Dr. Stough was finally con-strained by Alabama, which "shut down the plasmapheresis centers in the middle of the epidemics and blocked Dr. Stough's efforts to start them up again." [76]

It is likely that the reason Dr. Stough stayed in business as long as he did was his use of persons considered expendable. If the hepati-tis epidemic had occurred in the public school system and young children had been dying "slowly and in very painful fashion," there would have been outrage and calls for swift action, followed by thorough investigations and prosecutions. Stough's work, however, happened in the grey world of prisons that held a shunned popula-tion. Public agencies argued that their jurisdiction stopped at the prison wall. For those few that still retained authority inside the walls, staff shortages became the excuse. One FDA official argued, "Our responsibility is not the direct supervision of the drug investi-gators. Our responsibility is to evaluate the data that come in to us. We can't be omnipotent or omniscient." Involvement from state authori-ties was no better. As an Alabama public health official said, "The state health department has no specific jurisdiction in the prisons." [77]

By the end of the decade, Dr. Austin Stough was out of the prison drug testing business, but he did not leave empty-handed; the mil-lions of dollars he made were a testament to his own questionable practices, pharmaceutical company self-interest, and the indifference of governmental and correctional officials to the misdeeds taking place in their own facilities.

Stough may have been one of the more egregious examples of physicians who, through their experiments, placed prisoners at risk. But all those who engaged in resarch programs shared the same myopic view of their test subjects: prisoners offered a means to an end. In the spring and summer of 1961, the public learned of large-scale hepatitis experiments at the Illinois State Penitentiary at Joliet, the site of "clinical tests" to "conquer one of the more serious infectious diseases"—infectious hepatitis.[78] Between 137 and 200 inmates participated in the five-year-long study under the guidance of Dr. Joseph D. Boggs, director of laboratories at Children's Memorial Hospital in Chicago and associate professor of pathology at the Northwestern University School of Medicine. Infectious hepatitis had been a growing problem in the late 1950s and early 1960s—there were 32,000 new cases in the United States in just the first 18 weeks of 1961, double the number of the year before—and researchers were stymied because "the forms of the virus that produce human hepatitis...have no effect on animals," thus precluding using animals for tests. Doctors said that treatment was "hampered," and it was "necessary to use human volunteers."[79] It was reported that although many prisoners became ill, doctors wanted to assure newsmen that "there were no fatalities" among the Joliet volunteers.

A year later, American citizens learned that medical science had discovered a cure, as well as a preventative for a particular strain of malaria. Not surprisingly, this "remarkable...success" was accomplished at the Atlanta Federal Penitentiary, the site of so many malaria experiments.[80] Dr. G. Robert Coatney of the National Institutes of Health said that the "new experimental drug" lasted nearly "10 times longer" than conventional malaria suppressives and had shown itself to be "an apparent cure" for the disease. Known as CI501, "the drug was developed by scientists at Parke, Davis & Co. of Ann Arbor, Michigan," and was tested on 50 inmates at the federal facility.

The *New York Times* was so impressed by the prisoners' contribution in this latest malaria study that they printed an unusual article enumerating the various inmate contributions to medical science over the years and called for similar research that would benefit the "prisoners themselves."[81] The article said it was "ironic" that inmates had participated in everything from syphilis to polio studies, and yet there was a "paucity of research" dealing with the causes of crime. "Our prison inmates," the article plaintively argued, "have done so much to contribute to research [that they now] deserve to have more research done on their problems."

One would be hard pressed to find any therapeutic programs for prisoners established at this time. What was established instead were more clinical trials, including another malaria study. The Stateville Penitentiary in Illinois began one more malaria experiment in 1962 that used more than 400 inmates in a four-year-long project that hoped to discover remedies to currently resistant strains of the tropical disease.[82]

Throughout the 1960s, prisons hosted a stream of less controversial experiments as well, including numerous common cold studies. Federal prisoners were used in a variety of experiments dealing with the transmission of "airborne particles" that contribute to coughing, sneezing, and more severe flu-like diseases.[83] In 1968 the "first of its kind" spray vaccine, reported to be "much more effective than vaccine conventionally injected," was tested on hundreds of state prisoners in Florida. According to the doctors at the University of Florida College of Medicine, the results "may foreshadow a new era in vaccines against respiratory infections, possibly including the common cold."[84] An additional strategy, Dr. Linus Pauling's claim that "large doses of vitamin C can prevent and cure the common cold," was closely examined by a research team at the University of Maryland. The Maryland study conducted "among 21 prisoner-volunteers,...showed no preventive or therapeutic effectiveness of vitamin C."[85] Another influenza study coordinated by the National Institute of Allergy and Infectious Diseases in Bethesda, Maryland, used inmates at the District of Columbia's Lorton Reformatory and the Maryland House of Corrections in Jessup, Maryland, to test a "live, temperature sensitive virus" to create a "live hybrid vaccine."[86] Believed to be the "first live vaccine for influenza in this country," researchers hoped the new vaccine would be adaptable to any new strain of flu that entered the country.

County penal facilities were also attractive to enterprising researchers: inmates generally did not ask a lot of questions, and physicians and pharmaceutical firms did not go out of their way to inform the test subjects. Recruitment notices usually adopted a shotgun approach, employing every attractive carrot to induce prisoner participation. One cheerful, cartoon-filled brochure for another malaria study—this time in Jackson County, Missouri—offered volunteers "additional food, ice cream, fruit juice, improved quarters, and a $50 honorarium."[87] In addition, upon the program's completion, participants were to be "awarded a diploma-sized Certificate of Merit suitable for framing, commending them for their display of social responsibility and unselfishness."

IX

Throughout the boom years of the 1960s, drug companies raced to acquire friendly relationships with doctors who had prison practices. Phase I studies were critical to the development of new pharmaceutical products and some companies were willing to invest sizable sums to enhance their existing prison testing programs. In 1964, Upjohn and Parke-Davis contributed more than a half million dollars to build a state-of-the-art laboratory inside the walls of the State Prison of Southern Michigan, at Jackson. Rated the world's largest walled penitentiary, enclosing 57 acres and over 4,100 inmates, Jackson was no stranger to drug experimentation. Parke-Davis had been testing there for 30 years and Upjohn for eight. In 1961, "Dr. Harold Upjohn broached the idea of company laboratories at the prison to Gus Harrison, director of the Michigan Board of Corrections."[88] They took the idea to the prison commission "with the argument that research labs could be considered an extension of prison work shops and other activities geared to rehabilitation of prisoners." Under the agreement between the drug companies and the prison board, "companies [were] training inmates to run the tests that [could] be handled in the prison labs." Such maneuvers saved the drug companies from hiring expensive doctors and medical technicians by substituting cheap and abundant inmate labor. In 1968, some of the inmates brought a lawsuit against the companies and the corrections department, alleging that the "companies are obtaining or have obtained hundreds of thousands of dollars worth of labor free."[89] Inmate workers were usually paid between 35 cents and $1.25 a day, depending on the work assignment. Even if workers double-shifted each day, their weekly pay would be a bare fraction of what those jobs commanded on the

outside. The lab contained "two 10-bed metabolic wards" and generally tested "anti-coagulants, analgesics, anesthetics, steroids, tranquilizers and deodorants." The new facility would allow them "to
test drugs that have never been tried on human subjects." These
Phase I tests concentrated on "the toxicity of a drug, rather than its
efficacy,"[90] but the inmate-volunteers often found the potential dangers of the tests less of a threat than daily survival in prison. Some
considered the Upjohn and Parke-Davis laboratories an "oasis in a
desert," a needed respite from the daily threats and occasional warfare that are part of prison life. Pat Duffy, Jr., for example, told an
inquiring panel that their concern over prison testing policies was
misplaced and terribly naive. With seven years served on a 30- to
50-year sentence, Duffy had this to say about prison life and participation in medical research:

> First of all you have to understand the philosophy of prison, and
> you can't do that unless you've been in prison. There's a lot of do-
> gooders that come in and take the ten dollar tour. But you don't
> know what it's all about. You don't have to walk in the yard. You
> don't have to have your neck on a ball-bearing so you can see 360
> degrees around so that you can protect your life.
>
> Upjohn and Parke-Davis in the minds of most prisoners, is one
> of the positive aspects of life in the prison. You go over there when
> you want to hide out a little bit, when you want to talk to people
> that are going to treat you half way decent.
>
> But when you look at prison life, you're looking at something
> completely different from what you have on the outside, a com-
> pletely different society. It's turned around. Out in the street,
> when you walk around, you say, Well, someone may knock me in
> the head and take my wallet. Someone may sneak up on me at
> night by my car and molest me. And you're right, someone might
> do that. But when you are walking around Jackson Prison, you
> have 300 jerks up there that you know have done something
> wrong. When you look at the guy next to you, he's in maximum
> security because he's already done something. You know he's
> capable of tearing your head off at any moment. So, Upjohn and
> Parke-Davis, far from being something that would be a detriment
> to me or my colleagues up there, is looked on almost like a chapel.
> We go to those tests, and it's pure enjoyment. The little bit of irri-
> tation that you might be exposed to on Phase I testing is nothing
> compared to the madness that goes on in the yard.[91]

The California Medical Facility at Vacaville used another approach to form connections among prisoners, pharmaceutical companies, and enterprising doctors. Specifically designed for men in need of psychiatric treatment, anywhere from one-third to two-thirds of its 1,500 inmates volunteered for the medical research program. As opposed to the Upjohn/Parke-Davis initiative, which was organized by two drug companies, the Vacaville operation was, as author Jessica Mitford described, "under the aegis of a shadowy outfit called the Solana Institute for Medical and Psychiatric Research (SIMPR)."[92] SIMPR, established as a nonprofit corporation under the state's charitable trust law, saw its income rise from $47,000 in 1963, its first year of business, to over a quarter of a million dollars by 1971.

Though supposedly "barred from receiving money from private business concerns," SIMPR's income was derived from physicians who received research grants. As Ms. Mitford discovered, "various researchers from neighboring University of California medical schools were merely a conduit for tax-exempt payments from giant pharmaceutical concerns, including Lederle, Wyeth, Dow Chemical, Roche, Abbott, and Smith Kline & French." And a brochure to potential customers that extolled the safety record of SIMPR's drug testing program emphasized that "the reservoir of volunteer subjects offers investigational possibilities not found elsewhere." But, SIMPR's safety record was not as sound as it claimed, as evidenced by a lawsuit that was settled out of court for $6,000 and revealed by Mitford.

Two of the key researchers in the 1962 experiment under question were Dr. William L. Epstein, chairman of the dermatology department at the University of California and Dr. Howard I. Maibach. Both physicians were educated in dermatology in the residency program at the University of Pennsylvania School of Medicine and had received their practical training in research at Holmesburg Prison under the tutelage of Dr. Albert M. Kligman. That early prison experience proved so inspirational, they tried to establish a similar research enterprise on the West Coast.

The plaintiff had been classified as psychotic and sent to Vacaville for psychiatric programming and treatment. He was also one of twenty inmates selected to undergo what Dr. Epstein called "pain tolerance studies" consisting of intramuscular injections of Varidase, a Lederle Laboratories product. The plaintiff claimed he was held by four prison trustees and "forcibly injected with the drug in both arms." Independent medical personnel confirmed he thereafter suffered a near fatal muscular disease that caused his weight to drop from 140 to 75 pounds. The steroids used to treat the muscular disease caused chronic stomach ulcers.

As Jessica Mitford showed, when prison experiments went awry and victims brought lawsuits, the paper trail seemed to evaporate and doctors claimed innocence of any participation or knowledge of Varidase. In fact, they claimed they "had never heard of" the drug. The experiment was established to monitor "pain and the fever...what we were looking for was pain, discomfort, aching in the arm. We were told [by Lederle that the subjects might also suffer] fever, malaise, and chills." Even though Epstein was the principle investigator in the experiment, he could not recall if he was present when the subjects were chosen or when they received the injections. The shots, in fact, were given by inmate nurses, as was common in such drug testing ventures. Epstein was an infrequent visitor to his testing program, showing up "once a week or once every two weeks." When the 20 test subjects complained of "sharp abdominal pains, cold chills, headaches," and more, particularly in the plaintiff's case, Dr. Epstein didn't hesitate. He wrote Lederle: "We are planning this week to try four more men and I am prepared to give them some steroids when the severe symptomatology starts."

As a preventive measure against future lawsuits, SIMPR adopted a consent form and waiver: "I hereby fully and forever release, acquit, and discharge" all state agencies involved, plus SIMPR, "from any and all liability which may accrue" from participation in the research project.

Ms. Mitford went on to illuminate several other questionable practices of the SIMPR researchers, including low inmate wage rates that allowed drug companies to obtain "some $7.8 million worth of research for their $787,000" investment, experimental protocols that were never brought before medical peer review committees, and less than vigorous FDA oversight. As one independent medical expert with "wide experience in human research" asked rhetorically:

> If the researchers really believe these experiments are safe for humans, why do they go to the prison for the subjects? Why don't they try them out in their own laboratories on students or other free world volunteers? Because they know the university would never permit this—and furthermore it would never enter their minds to do these things to people they associate with in daily life. They make a distinction between people they think of as social equals or colleagues and men behind bars, whom they regard as less than human.[93]

While the Vacaville experiments were taking place, the federal government, through the Atomic Energy Commission, was funding a decade-long series of radiation experiments on Oregon and Washington State prison inmates. "The tests were designed to help determine how much radiation U.S. astronauts could bear during space flights" and were closely watched by National Aeronautics and Space Administration scientists.[94] Participation was voluntary and inmates were given small cash payments, but they had to undergo risky radiation exposure to their testicles. Harold Bibeau, at the time, a 23-year-old inmate, was told to lie down in "a coffin-like box and lower his testicles into water."[95] Researchers then exposed them to a dose of radiation equivalent to 20 modern diagnostic X-rays. "It was warm down there," recalls Bibeau, nearly 30 years after the experiment, "like I have been laying in the sun for too long." Testicles are especially sensitive to radiation; even slight chromosomal damage can lead to infertility, testicular cancer, and birth defects. After the radiation treatment, Bibeau had to provide urine and semen samples, and undergo periodic biopsies.

In all, the testicles of more than 130 Oregon and Washington prisoners were irradiated. The radiation experiments were halted in the early 1970s, but survivors are still coming forward to describe their health maladies. Many complain of prostate cancer, vision loss, vascular problems, and sexual identity questions.

"I took part in the tests and now I'm in a lot of pain," says Philip King, a subject in 1969 when a state prison inmate in Salem,

Oregon.[96] The 54-year old King complains of groin pains so severe that he sometimes has trouble sitting down. Another former Oregon inmate, Robert Garrison, recalls repeated radiation exposures over several weeks in the late 1960s and now has to contend with "persistent rashes and a painful lump on his testicles."[97]

In 1976, a group of former Oregon inmates brought a lawsuit, but detailed information about the experiments was not revealed until December 1994, when a 14-member committee was appointed by the White House to investigate the issue of federal radiation tests on humans. A number of medical researchers who oversaw the experiments declined to appear at the federal hearings. Energy Secretary Hazel O'Leary, who brought the issue to the attention of the American public in 1993, was "charged with determining whether financial compensation, medical tests, or other kinds of follow-up should be given to the participants."[98] According to some estimates, almost half of the prison test subjects have died.

X

Despite the increasing pressure on administrators in the field of human research to conform to new government mandates during the late 1960s and early 1970s, project protocols show researchers continued to view prison volunteers as the perfect population for scientific study—cheap, available, and confined. The rubella project in Petersburg (Virginia) was under the direction of Dr. John L. Sever of the National Institutes of Health, and used men between 21 and 28 years old who were willing to expose themselves to a "progressive, uniformly fatal disease which involves a chronic...measles infection of the central nervous system."[99] For their 16 weeks of participation, $20 was credited to the volunteer's account, which he could use "for making purchases at the Reformatory store" or have it "available for him at the time of release."

Lompoc (California) and Stafford (Arizona) were holding weightlessness experiments, simulated by extended bed rest, for the National Aeronautic and Space Administration. Participation in this study paid considerably better, $50 per month and an extra $50 for completing the test. Organized at the U.S. Public Health Service

Hospital in San Francisco, the experiment ran between 1969 and 1975 and was designed to better understand "the effects of total bed rest on heart, blood vessels and bones."[100] Apparently, NASA was also "keenly interested" in this project since they hoped to gain valuable clues "from bed rest" about "the changes of weightlessness in space." By late 1969, "more than 50 volunteers had taken part," with a half dozen having remained in bed more than six months. No one appeared to suffer "any ill effects," but by the early 1970s test subjects were being forced to wear compression suits, and endure endless blood and calcium tests, numerous radioactive isotope injections, and the normal bone and muscle loss caused during prolonged bed rest. As usual, a consent form had been signed by the participants, but by this time enough scrutiny and criticism of such practices had been leveled that the form stated that it "shall not be construed as a release of NASA from any future liability."

By 1973, the pressure on state and federal penal systems that performed medical research on prisoners had reached critical mass. Critics of the practice were growing rapidly in number and their criticisms were increasingly hostile. On a regular basis, American physicians doing clinical trials in prisons had to confront allusions to Nazi-like medical experiments. Jessica Mitford fired a rhetorical broadside at proponents of using prisoners as research subjects with the publication of *Kind and Usual Punishment*, a powerful and sobering indictment of punishment in America. Mitford devoted a revealing chapter, entitled "Cheaper Than Chimpanzees," to prison experimentation, placing particular emphasis on America's departure from the spirit of Nuremberg in its use of prisoners as research subjects. As she boldly stated, the Nuremberg Code, "if observed would end altogether the practice of using prisoners as subjects." She asked how American prisoners "stripped of their civil rights" when they enter the gates, "subjected to years or decades of confinement," could be free agents capable of "exercising freedom of choice?"[101] Coming on the heels of the bloody prison riot at Attica, in which several dozen inmates and guards lost their lives, the general public was all too willing to believe the cruel and unusual conditions that Mitford described in U.S. prisons.

Ms. Mitford was also one of the prominent witnesses to testify before a U.S. Senate subcommittee, chaired by Senator Edward Kennedy, investigating a broad range of human experimentation issues.[102] The hearing came on the heels of revelations about the Tuskegee Syphilis Study; however, considerable time was devoted to prisoner experimentation. In addition to scholars, journalists, and ex-offenders, who painted a negative picture of prison research, were representatives of the Pharmaceutical Manufacturers Association, which argued that prisoners did have free will, informed consent, the right to participate in drug studies, and that any governmental intrusion into such practices would result in dire consequences for the industry.

All across the country, however, newspaper articles and editorials began to discuss the increasingly controversial issue of human experimentation in prisons. For example, under the title "Jailed Guinea Pigs," a *New York Times* editorial argued that the "basic question is whether incarcerated people who enter programs involving cholera, typhoid fever, and smallpox can ever truly be said to have volunteered."[103] For this newspaper and many others like it, the "question of coercion, both overt and covert," was the centerpiece of the debate: could imprisoned individuals truly give consent? A growing number of people were saying no, and prison systems that had once hosted human research began to terminate their programs. Allyn R. Sielaff, commissioner of corrections in Illinois, called experiments on prisoners "immoral and unethical" and ordered a halt to the system's famed Stateville malaria project after 29 years of research.[104]

In the summer of 1974, responding to protests in the Maryland State prison system, Congressman Parren Mitchell introduced H.R. 16160, "*A Bill To Limit the Use of Prison Inmates in Medical Research*," which focused on shutting down experimentation in federal prisons.[105] The bill also tried to affect state penal facilities by calling for the end of all such endeavors in those state systems that received federal monies. The bill died in the 93rd Congress, but upon reintroduction as H.R. 3603 the following term, hearings were held on the legislation and philosophical combatants representing both sides squared off.[106] Emotions had become so heightened by this point that some who believed they had "led...the struggle to stop the exploitation of prisoners in medical research" felt "black ball[ed]" when they were not invited to address the committee.[107] One issue activist, for example, denounced the prominent position given "white professionals representing the interests of Black people" and saw the hearing as a continuation of "racist and elitist" government policies. At the hearing, one of the most surprising pieces of testimony came from Dr. John D. Arnold, a long-time champion of prison research who began his career at Stateville Penitentiary. Arnold had concluded that scientific investigators and drug companies could continue their work without the use of prisoners.[108] His conclusion was unexpected; for years prison research adherents had been predicting doom if prisoners were precluded from volunteering for pharmaceutical testing. Many believed the real reason for the gloomy forecast was economic; free-world volunteers would be more expensive. Just a year earlier, during another congressional hearing on the need for greater controls in human experimentation, Senator Ted Kennedy had this exchange with the president of the Pharmaceutical Manufacturers Association:

> SEN. KENNEDY: Your position is you couldn't get other citizens in the community, even given the financial remuneration, to undertake this type discipline?
> MR. STETLER: I can't say "couldn't" because it has not been tried.
> SEN. KENNEDY: It has or has not been tried?
> MR. STETLER: It has not been tried.
> SEN. KENNEDY: Why has it not been tried?
> MR. STETLER: I suppose because it is too difficult.
> SEN. KENNEDY: You haven't tried yet? How do you know it is difficult?
> MR. STETLER: You get back to the other points I mentioned earlier. When you have others available, you use them.
> SEN. KENNEDY: Is that because it is cheaper?
> MR. STETLER: It is cheaper.[109]

The Director of the Bureau of Prisons, Norman A. Carlson, began to spend an increasing portion of his time answering the questions of concerned federal lawmakers and testifying before them on Capitol Hill about the scope of human experimentation in federal prisons. In a January 1974 letter, Senator Sam Ervin, Jr., requested answers to dozens of questions, such as, "How extensive is the use of prisoners in biomedical or behavioral research projects?...What methods are used to secure volunteers for experiments conducted in the prisons?" and "Are there any system-wide standards or rules pertaining to research?"[110] Ervin's four-page, single-spaced letter to Carlson requesting detailed answers to 47 specific questions was more than a warning shot across the prison system's bow; it demonstrated a growing certainty that human experimentation in correctional institutions raised serious ethical questions, had problematic policy consequences, and fostered public concern. Ervin concluded his letter by stating "that research involving human subjects is essential to the future of medicine and thus to the human race. I feel equally strongly, however, the concern for the rights of the individual must assume the highest priority in any consideration of such experimentation."

Carlson was now communicating his "serious doubts about the ability of prisoners to volunteer for any form of medical research" and gradually curtailed the prison system's existing experimentation programs.[111] This decision satisfied interested legislators and concerned administration officials, but worried medical operatives dependent upon the prison system's supply of cheap and willing test subjects for their experiments. In a memo to the deputy attorney general, Director Carlson mentioned he had "received an irate call from Dr. Robert Dupont of NIMH" after the *Washington Post* made public the plans to phase out the use of federal prisoners at the Addiction Research Center.[112] The doctor believed the prison bureau "had reneged on an earlier commitment" concerning the project's phase-out. Others in the medical research community were also concerned about the loss of research subjects. Some had national reputations and were not hesitant to speak out. Dr. Albert Sabin, developer of the polio vaccine and the director of "hundreds of prisoners" as test subjects in Chillicothe, Ohio, claimed that a prison was one of the few areas where "a stable, long-time permanent study group" could be established for medical research.[113] He added that participation in research often gives the prisoners a sense of worth, some money, and the hope for an early release. Dr. Franz J. Inglefinger, editor of the highly respected *New England Journal of Medicine*, said a halt to such research would do severe damage to medical research, particularly for the "poor" who are most in need of it.

Interestingly, some of the most ardent supporters of the existing system and staunch opponents of governmental intrusion were the prisoners themselves. "It's unfair. I have a right to do what I want with myself," said Michael Filip, 31, a veteran of nearly two dozen experiments and, at that time, part of a $300-a-month "heart regulating drug study" at a Michigan prison.[114] The depth of prisoner support came as quite a shock to many members of the newly formed National Commission for the Protection of Human Subjects of Biomedical and Behavioral Research, an advisory panel of bioethical experts, that traveled to the Upjohn/Parke-Davis testing site at the state prison in southern Michigan. Overwhelmingly, the prisoners were opposed to the termination of the program; it was clear the money and other rewards were important to them. The commission's recommendations did not entirely close off the possibility of continued prison testing, but its stipulations for general prison improvement as a prerequisite for experimentation were too onerous, if not impossible, for any penal system hoping to continue the embattled practice.[115]

By this time, however, most correctional administrators, including Carlson, had had enough of the growing prison experimentation controversy and they strongly encouraged termination of such programs. The last vestige of federal inmate testing, the relationship with the Addiction Research Center, was on its death bed. "I firmly believe," Carlson wrote, "that we should get out of the project as soon as possible."[116] He also reinforced his memo by enclosing the recently passed resolution of the American Correctional Association calling for "the abandonment of all such projects." By June 1975, only 12 state prison systems were hosting medical experiments, and on March 1, 1976, Carlson announced the end of medical research on federal prisoners.[117]

During the course of 1976, one commission after another recommended the termination of prison medical experiments. Opposition to the controversial practice was now overwhelming. This "revolt," was fueled by the confluence of both scientific and social forces. They combined a new skepticism "about the fruits of scientific research" (the nuclear threat, chemical and pesticide pollution) and "rights-oriented movements" driven by women, minorities, mental health advocates, and others entering the policy arena.[118] "We don't want to kill science," said M. Carl Holman, president of the National Urban Coalition, "but we don't want science to kill, mangle, and abuse us."[119] Holman's organization had just sponsored the first National Minority Conference on Human Experimentation, which, not surprisingly, recommended "a moratorium on research involving prisoners...and the banning of all biomedical research and experimentation on inmates of prisons and jails." Conference members argued that minority groups, including the poor, the mentally infirm, and blacks, "were consistently exploited in research" and a national organization had to be established "to see that justice is done."

A modicum of prisoner experimentation continued, some into the 1980s, but for the most part what had become a controversial and odious research practice was effectively over. After a lengthy and tortured process, the Food and Drug Administration finally stated that clinical investigations for research purposes "may not involve prisoners as subjects."[120]

In prison after prison, and state after state, researchers with their scientific protocols and expensive laboratory equipment were sent packing. In some cases, research physicians departed before they were asked; experimentation with prisoners had become just too difficult. What was once a lucrative growth industry in medicine had become a victim of its own excesses and changes in community ethics. America's medical establishment was finally made to observe the decades-old Nuremberg Code. Physicians retained a prestigious place in society, but their past insularity became increasingly challenged as additional players joined medical and scientific decision making. Scientific advancement could no longer depend on vulnerable populations as raw material. Pharmaceutical companies continued to develop successful products by testing new drugs on volunteers, but never as cheaply and as effortlessly as when

America provided an open-door policy to its penal institutions. A generation after American judges sentenced Gerhard Rose and his Nazi colleagues in the Palace of Justice, the Nuremberg Code took up residence in America.

Part Three

CRUEL AND UNUSUAL EXPERIMENTS

Four

"The Walls Seemed To Be Breathing."

I

Johnnie Williams, a former Holmesburg inmate, remembers the Army trailers well. Williams's numerous arrests over four decades enabled him to participate in many of Dr. Kligman's experiments, and he became one of Holmesburg Prison's most persistent and active experimental recruits. But the battery of tests he underwent in the trailers stand out. Williams, a powerfully built, dark-complexioned man, who has lost the threatening swagger of his youth and now tries to hide a slight limp, believes he was used for a number of mind-disabling experiments including at least two LSD tests. "I had some really bad experiences in those trailers," says Williams in an interview.[1]

Johnnie Williams was no stranger to criminal activity. Born and raised on the mean ghetto streets of North Philadelphia, his father, a construction worker, and his mother, a housewife, tried to give their only child "everything [he] ever wanted." Williams says he had a "good home life...but I had no brothers or sisters so I wanted to be accepted by the gang." When the local Valley Gang discovered he "could fight," Williams became an important member. All through junior high and high school in the 1950s, he spent considerable time in turf battles. At age 18, Williams stole a car and was arrested for the first time; he was convicted and sentenced to two years probation. When he violated parole in 1957, he was consigned to Holmesburg Prison and served nearly five months. He stayed clear of the research program because the "tests looked scary."

In 1963, Williams was back in Holmesburg on a burglary charge and was less opposed to the experiments. He "needed bail money" so he volunteered for a "patch test." One test led to another; Williams had discovered a way to earn money, and soon he was open to just about any experimental venture that paid well. Young, strong, and seemingly impervious to physical injury, Williams believed the experiments were at most a minor nuisance always off-set by the attractive pay. "I did lipstick, surgical equipment, toothpaste, cosmetics, peyote cigarettes, and a lot of other stuff," says Williams with a certain amount of pride.

A generally loud, gregarious, whimsical man, with deep-set eyes, Williams carries his hefty frame from chore to chore outside the stark cement walls of Graterford State Prison in Southeastern Pennsylvania. His playful demeanor, prominence as a cook, and long years of imprisonment have made him a familiar character at the penitentiary where the Holmesburg experiments are a well-known phenomenon. Many of the older prisoners at the institution either endured the experiments themselves or know somebody who did. The old-timers all point to Williams as an authority on the tests.

He tells of discolorations on his forearm from "a microwave light" that burned him; exposure to "sulfuric acid and carbolic acid"; diet milkshake tests at which he was "caught cheating" and "kicked off"; putting his arm in solutions for "one hour over 30 straight days" until his "skin was like leather"; and "acid" rubbed on his testicles while a "tin cup [was] placed underneath to catch the blistered skin....We got $3 for that test," he says disdainfully.

"The sweat test," as Williams refers to it, placed inmates in an overheated chamber, after which their armpit glands were cut for examination. In another test, sutures were made in his body "to see if they would dissolve," and in keloid tests, "some stuff [was] injected in his back" and then removed bit by bit. He claims to have had "part of a cadaver" implanted in his "back to see if it would grow," but after a couple of days his "body rejected it." Williams recalls participating in tests of Hong Kong flu, poison ivy, and poison oak. The patch tests, he says, were the easiest to endure because each time he returned to his cell, he, like other inmates, would "hang the patch on the wall."

There were a few tests that even Williams declined. He remembers "guys with big things attached to their faces and foreheads," in what inmates called "the Cyclops Test." "I didn't do that, I was afraid of it....[and] I never did the liver and lung biopsies...they looked too scary and dangerous." He describes "needles about a foot long" and shivers at the memory. "I used to sneak [in] and read the papers" (meaning the experimental protocols) that doctors left in the research unit, says Williams with a proud grin. As head cook, he "sold swag [contraband] sandwiches to the U of P personnel" and they rewarded him with the most desirable tests—those that held the least risk, but garnered a lot of money. "Guys would let [me] know what was really damaging and wouldn't let [me] take the test." He followed such valuable advice when offered. Those less connected, or more in need of cash, were fair game for the most risky experiments.

He recalls other experiments with laughter, and recounts the deodorant study. After a thorough wash with soap and water, the inmates applied a brand of deodorant and went out in the yard to play a vigorous game of handball. They returned to line up in front of female inspectors who had been brought especially to smell the inmates' armpits. Another test that amused Williams was the fungus experiment (what he thought was a footwear test). Prisoners were made to wear galoshes, and occasionally boots, for five straight days. The boots were taped on and the inmates even slept in them.

Johnnie Williams is also pretty sure who sponsored these tests. He rattles off high-powered corporate names like Squibb, Merck, Sharpe and Dohme, Proctor and Gamble, Parke-Davis, and Helena Rubenstein. He became so addicted to the money that he claims to have participated in "ten or twelve tests at one time." He displays his abdominal scars from various biopsies as matter-of-factly as a veteran shows his war wounds. (Prison veterans view surviving the prison experience as no less an accomplishment than surviving front-line military duty.) Money was an important survival tool. Patch tests, milkshakes, and biopsies could bring anywhere from a few dollars to $30, $40, or $50 at a time. Special tests like the Army experiments brought in "between $700 and $800," what Williams claims he was paid for his first Army test. Because of the extraordinary financial rewards he went back "four or five times," even though his experience with chemical warfare agents was less than positive.

"I used the money to make bail," says Williams. Holmesburg held many men who, like himself, were indicted and awaiting trial; under Philadelphia's 10 percent cash bail system, $5,000 bail meant the inmate needed $500 to get back on the streets. In the 1950s and 1960s, considerably less than $500 could free a number of low-risk, low-bail prisoners awaiting their days in court. Even in the early 1970s, inmates could be found trying to scrape up small amounts of cash to meet a low bail figure. Although Williams made a lot of money over the years as a willing and eager test subject, he is now angry at the experimenters and critical of his own short-sighted thinking. In his defense, he argues that "we were never told what was going on. We never had witnesses or a receipt for anything [we] signed."

Participation in the riskier experiments, such as the Army's incapacitation studies, brought the greatest financial rewards, but only for the stout of heart. For those inside the walls of Holmesburg—inmates and guards alike—the Army trailers represented something different, even eerie; a place where "they messed with your mind." Williams recounts that after his recruitment and "screening"—an extensive physical and psychological examination—he was taken to the trailers, where he was injected with a solution in the back of the arm. "Almost immediately I felt affected. I couldn't control myself and told them to get this shit out of me." He recalls hallucinating: "I'd be playing cards and all of a sudden the cards were gone. It scared me."

On one memorable occasion, Johnnie Williams "acted so badly" they had to give him an "antidote" and place him under close observation for several weeks. The memories of the incident are still fresh. Williams remembers being placed in a small, padded cell in one of the trailers and staring at the video and audio equipment located near the ceiling. As the effects of the injection grew stronger, he became captivated by the camera staring down at him, heard pleasant music coming out of it, and a short time later began to "see the damn notes come out of the lens." As, one at a time, they fell toward him, he felt he could almost reach out and grab them. The tranquil experience intrigued him and he enjoyed the sounds.

In the midst of his delusional rapture, Williams caught a glimpse of "McCluney," a medical technician, staring at him through the small square plexiglass window that allowed University of Pennsylvania testing personnel to observe the behavior of the experimental subjects. "I went off," says Williams. "I pulled the toilet bowl off the cell floor and threw it against the wall and then tore the cell door off the wall." To the relief of everyone in attendance, his destructive rampage ended at the door. As Dr. James Ketchum, a physician with the experiment, recalls: "I was pretty sure he would be menacing. He was a monster of a man, 250 pounds of muscle. He blew the door right off the hinges and they were pretty solid, well-built trailers. I was standing there pretty stunned. He said: "'Doc, I think I'd like to have an antidote to this stuff now.' I was gratified he was so well behaved because he could have done a lot of damage."[2]

Williams remembers his anger dissipating quickly once he discarded the door and reached the hallway of the trailer. "They let me go wherever I wanted to go and they just followed me. It seemed like forever." He believes he was "kept in another cell for two weeks" to recover from his "bad reaction" and when released wore the same identification badge described by Al Zabala. It read: "Please excuse this inmate's behavior. He can't think or act in a coherent manner and is part of the U.S. Army testing program." Williams recalls walking all over the institution, even the center control area, in a trance-like state and no one was allowed to touch him. According to Williams, if he caused any disruption, medical personnel from the University of Pennsylvania research unit were instructed to bring him back to H Block or the adjoining Army trailers.

Today, Johnnie Williams speaks calmly about his experiences in the Army tests. The blackouts and sleepless nights have ended, although his many scars and skin discolorations remind him of his recklessness. He is clear, however, about one thing: his personality took a dramatic turn after the Army tests. He claims he went from being a small-time hood before the tests to a violent criminal afterwards. Williams says, "I did small crimes, nonviolent crimes, things like burglary, car theft, and petty thievery....I had been a guy who tried to avoid arguments, but after the tests...I got very quick tempered and got into a lot of fights....The crimes got worse...I went from petty thievery and busting into cars, to shootings, and assaults. I had major problems after the tests. [They] made me violent. I did things to provoke people....I never did that before."

II

The pursuit of advances in chemical warfare brought the Army trailers to Holmesburg Prison. From the point that Woodrow Wilson authorized the Chemical Warfare Service (CAWS) during World War I, human experimentation was an integral part of the U.S. Army's chemical warfare operations. By 1922, CAWS had created a division to conduct research into providing defenses against chemical agents developed by other countries.

The threat of World War II once again triggered the need for antidotes to chemical weapons—antidotes that could be tested on a large source of volunteers. In 1942, the Secretary of War granted formal authority to recruit volunteer subjects in chemical warfare experiments. By the following year, CAWS was given responsibility for all medical research into chemical warfare and toxic agents.

In the early 1950s, the Armed Forces Medical Policy Council took up the issue of using humans in medical experiments, and stipulated that they had to be volunteers. CAWS, which had now become the Chemical Corps, had developed a human experimentation game plan, but lacked the key ingredient of an adequate pool of volunteers. The dilemma was rectified in 1955 by the decision to use enlisted men stationed at Army facilities near Edgewood Arsenal, Maryland. In conjunction with this initiative, it was determined "that voluntary consent of each subject was absolutely essential...subjects would be thoroughly informed of all procedures...of what might be expected as a result of each test,...and [of] the volunteer's right to determine whether he desired to participate in a given experiment."[3] In the fall of 1959, approval was granted to conduct research on incapacitating chemical warfare agents.

An incapacitating agent acts on the nervous system and affects, either rapidly or over a period of time, an individual's performance and behavior, but does not inflict permanent injury or death. For the military, incapacitation means the inability to perform one's military assignment. The American military was looking for more sophisticated, less crude and terrible, chemical agents than the mustard, phosgene, and chlorine gases that had killed and maimed hundreds of thousands of soldiers during World War I. The Geneva Convention of 1925 had placed a ban on the use of chemical weapons, and while the United States supported the goals of the declaration, we did not sign it; instead, the United States continued to develop and stockpile various nerve agents.

Several countries were appropriating large sums to chemical weapon research, in particular the United States and the Soviet Union. Each feared the other's presumed triumphs in this still-developing science of psychopharmacology that fostered a comprehensive exploration of incapacitants. The goal of discovering an incapacitating agent that could "produce temporary military ineffectiveness without permanent injury or death" was a difficult one, since few pharmacological substances seemed capable of performing this dual role. One promising area appeared to be "comprised almost entirely of compounds whose major site of action is within the central nervous system."[4]

In America, thousands of soldiers volunteered as test subjects, and the Chemical Corps established the recruitment procedure that would later be followed at Holmesburg. Enlisted men at various Army installations were given a briefing that usually included a film and handouts. Generally 10 to 20 percent of the enlisted men expressed interest in the program, were asked to complete a medical and psychological personal history, and took the Minnesota Multiphase Personality Inventory (MMPI). Usually, no more than 100 out of 400 to 600 volunteers were chosen and assigned to a one- or two-month tour of duty at Edgewood Arsenal. The men received a small monetary allowance of generally less than $2 a day, and were granted light duty and free weekends. The volunteers were described as "above average in physical and mental qualifications, [having] good behavior records and normal MMPI's."[5]

The Army claims that it relied on the Nuremberg and Helsinki guidelines in the studies it performed on volunteers, although they acknowledge that this was not clearly articulated in official memoranda until the mid-1960s. They also claim that, at an early stage in their testing, they adopted written consent forms that became more sophisticated as the years passed. To protect the volunteers' welfare under the varied tests it planned, the Army says it built a comprehensive medical staff that included physicians trained in psychiatry, internal medicine, anesthesiology, cardiology, surgery, dermatology, ophthalmology, neurology, and other specialties. A high percentage of these doctors were serious, research-oriented scientists who went on to distinguished academic careers at leading universities around the country.

For a 20-year period, from approximately 1955 to 1975, the Army conducted experiments to learn how specific chemicals affected humans. Among the most common of the 254 chemicals tested were "acutely toxic anticholinesterase chemicals: incapacitating agents, which included the glycolates, atropine-like anticholinergic compounds of which BZ (3-quinuclidinyl benzilate) is a prototype; the indoles, represented by EA 1729 (LSD-25); the cannabinols, or marijuana-like compounds; and the sedative, or tranquilizer, group."[6] The Army was most interested in testing psychological or behavioral drugs—known by some as psychochemicals. The drug group deliriants, as opposed to stimulants, depressants, and psychedelics, includes drugs that have many utilitarian purposes at low dosages on a clinical level but that at higher doses can cause severe delirium characterized by hallucination, confusion, and disorganized speech and behavior. The deliriants became the centerpiece of their testing from the mid- to late 1960s. Particularly interesting were a subgroup known as anticholinergics, which include atropine and scopolamine. Derived from Jimson (loco) weed and Mandrake root, the anticholinergics affect the central nervous system, vision, muscle reflexes, and heart rate as well as other organs and bodily functions. Scopolamine is about sevenfold more potent than atropine, but is shorter acting. An additional drug, 3-quinuclidinyl benzilate, or BZ, is stronger yet (roughly 25 times the impact of atropine) and has subsequently "gained a reputation as an exceptionally potent and dangerous drug."[7] Slow to take effect but long in duration, BZ has a number of characteristics that the military found advantageous, and they sought more documentation through human trials. According to a 1975 Army inspector general's report, revised figures show that more than

7,000 military volunteers took part in the Edgewood Arsenal drug tests and more than 1,000 civilians participated in similar studies at universities and hospitals on contract to the Army.[8]

III

The question naturally arises, with tens of thousands of military personnel available and an apparently more than adequate number of soldiers actively enrolled in tests, why did it become necessary to switch to university physicians and prison inmates? The answer apparently involves a combination of entrepreneurial zeal at the university level and the Army's desire for validation of its test procedures and results by university-based academic authorities.

Destruction of valuable paperwork and the unwillingness of many individuals to discuss their roles in the prison experiments make it hard to arrive at definitive answers. But important clues arise from the few remaining documents and the recollections of some experimental operatives. According to one formerly confidential Army document, authored by James Ketchum, David Kitzes, and Herbert Copelan, the Holmesburg Prison connection developed in the following manner. In the early 1960s, the Army was studying a variety of belladonna-like compounds that revealed in humans a considerable variation in the time of onset and duration.[9] Scopolamine, for example, produced effects within minutes but lasted only a few hours, while a benzilate produced peak central nervous system effects at about eight hours and had a delirious effect for 24 to 72 hours. According to this document, two accidental exposures precipitated the research at Holmesburg. In the first, a pharmacologist conducting intravenous studies of 3-quinuclidinyl cyclopentylphenylglycolate (EA 3167) in dogs accidentally injected a small amount of the compound, subcutaneously, into his thumb. A couple of days later he was brought into the emergency room in a delirious state and was admitted to the experimental ward for observation. The use of an intravenous antidote reversed the delirium, but it returned when medication was interrupted. After two weeks he was released, but irritability and memory problems remained and required an extended readjustment to his job. After six months the doctor appeared fully recovered.

In the second case, a young chemist had a similar accident and required hospitalization. After he was released, intellectual tasks proved difficult for months. In six months, he appeared to have recovered fully from his exposure and seemed to suffer no lasting psychological or intellectual impairment.

Because of the "unusually prolonged effects" of this substance, it was decided that the compound deserved greater study; Edgewood, however, lacked adequate testing capacity. Moreover, because of the potency of the chemical agent, a test subject needed to remain under observation longer than a soldier's 2-month assignment to Edgewood. In 1964, anxious to find a university-centered research facility along the eastern seaboard, the Army engaged the University of Pennsylvania and Holmesburg Prison inmates to find the minimum effective dose (MED) of EA 3167. Initially, 19 healthy male volunteers between the ages of 22 and 37 were selected for the experiments; the inmates had been chosen on the basis of the Army's usual battery of tests and interviews. Doctors measured heart rate, blood pressure, body temperature, pupil size, and respiration and compiled "a chest film, complete hemogram and urinalysis, electrocardiogram, and liver and renal function tests." Only inmates with at least six months of their sentence remaining were allowed to participate to ensure "adequate follow-up testing."

Cognitive performance influenced the prisoner's payment. A battery of tests, including the Wechsler Adult Intelligence Scale (WAIS), Draw-a-Person Test, Bender-Gestalt, Thematic Apperception Test, and the Harris-Lingo Subscales of the MMPI, was administered "to most subjects shortly before...drug administration,...[then again] after two weeks, four weeks, and [finally] six months." In addition, the Number Facility Test, a three-minute speed accuracy test, was used serially during the test period to monitor cognitive performance. Subjects received 2 cents for each correct answer during the trial baseline period, and 3 cents after having received the drug. The report stated that "previous work had shown that this schedule of reward maintains a high level of motivation in this population." According to a former test monitor, the financial rewards were not the *best* motivator, but the *only* motivator. "We never tried to appeal to their sense of patriotism or altruism," says Lawrence Byrne. "We told them this was a test you could make some money on."[10]

Hired in 1966 as a "psychologist technician" to facilitate the Army studies, Larry Byrne was a recent college graduate hoping to develop a career in psychology. He recalls the protocols as "very complete and specific," but he "never knew what chemicals were being used" because they were identified only by "numerically designated codes." Much of his job involved making sure that a "pool of subjects [was] ready" at all times. There were "long periods [when] we did no testing, but continued to screen people and keep an updated pool of subjects." Periodically, he would be told: "'I think you're gonna have an agent next week. Get your people ready.'" Byrne says that because the Army "wanted people who would be there for awhile," they "looked for lifers and those serving long terms."

As with all the Army experiments, the test subjects were given the chemical agent as a single intramuscular injection in the morning following a light breakfast. Dosages varied, but most injections of EA 3167 ran from 2.4 ug/kg to 3.4 ug/kg; observations were recorded hourly for six hours, then every two hours for the next six hours, and then at four-hour intervals.

Again according to the report, the test results showed a wide variation. Some subjects who had been given higher doses appeared "relatively unaffected," while a few remained delirious for up to two weeks. One subject, the most seriously affected, required doses of physostigmine repeated over 14 days to "prevent episodes of confused and uncooperative behavior."[11] "Hallucinations were common to almost half the group and tended to be more frequent and longer lasting in those receiving the highest doses. Cognitive performance was "clearly impaired in most subjects." The peak effect occurred between 12 and 24 hours and the drug's duration lasted anywhere from 48 hours to 21 days.

A later report reviewing the EA 3167 study discussed such physiologic results as altered heart rate, and blood pressure, the impact of minimum incapacitating doses on 50 percent of a given population (ID-50), and the duration of severe and mild effects. The study review also included several criticisms of the experimenters. The report pointed out that although the test volunteers reportedly showed no variation in pupil size, "observer error...seems to have been considerable, judging from the wide fluctuations in consecutive estimates by the technicians on duty."[12] Furthermore, the report's analysis of the long-term effects of the compound was incomplete because of "personnel turnover and delay in obtaining a qualified clinical psychologist."

The report confirmed what the exposed workers had demonstrated: EA 3167 was "exceptionally long-acting and highly potent."[13] In addition, the prisoners demonstrated a series of residual symptoms including "irritability, memory impairment, insomnia, blurred vision, and difficulty in concentrating." Although the doctors concluded that all measurable psychopathology on intellectual deficit resolved after six months, except in "one or more individuals," they allowed a variable. "Since the population from which the subjects were drawn is known to have a high incidence of psychopathological reactions not associated with identifiable stress, the flare-up of symptoms in a few subjects is difficult to interpret." In other words, the effects suffered by some of the inmates were due either to the drug or to the personality of the prisoner being tested.

Completed in 1975, "EA 3167: Effects in Man," was one of many experimental protocols that the University of Pennsylvania and Holmesburg Prison performed for the U.S. Army.

IV

According to a 1975 inspector general's report, the Army awarded six separate contracts to the University of Pennsylvania.[14] The initial contract in 1951 was entitled "Study of Chemical Warfare Casualties in Man" and was a laboratory study only. The next contract was designed to study the "Influence of Morphine and Demerol on the Respiratory Response of Man." Although approximately 40 volunteers" were engaged in the drug tests, the contract does "not reveal the source of these volunteers or any evidence regarding the screening, selection, or execution of volunteer agreements. In the early 1960s, the third and fourth contracts were signed. They dealt with the "Evaluation in Animals and Man, Drug and Drug Mixtures Intended for Use in Preventing or Treating Chemical Warfare Casualties." Apparently, 10 volunteers received scopolamine, atropine, and morphine. Once again, there is no information about the origin of the volunteers, the selection process, or medical preparations for the experiments.

The fifth and sixth contracts, executed in 1964, covered experiments on the "Threshold Doses in Humans and Evaluation of Drugs in Man." They identify the source of experimental volunteers as 320 inmates of Holmesburg Prison. The three-year study was designed to test 16 different chemical agents including ditran, atropine, scopolamine, and various experimental glycolate agents. The report defines glycolates as incapacitating because they interfere with "muscarinic functions (that is, the activation of smooth muscle and secretory glands) and the central nervous system functions of acetylcoline; they also depress or inhibit nervous activity,...cause delirium,...physical incoordination, blurred vision, inhibition of sweating and salivation, rapid heart rate, elevated blood pressure, increased body temperatures and at high doses, vomiting, prostration, and stupor or coma. The onset time may be minutes or hours or days."[15]

The inspector general's report also included a "contract chart" listing in alphabetical order all of the institutions that performed investigative drug studies for the Army from the early 1950s to the early 1970s.[16] Forty-eight separate contracts are listed, the bulk of them (29) awarded to 12 universities including the University of Washington, Baylor, Tulane, Johns Hopkins, New York University, and the Universities of Utah and Indiana. Many of the schools received hundreds of thousands of dollars for their efforts. The University of Colorado, for example, earned over $175,000 in the 1950s for three separate contracts on the "Investigation and Testing of Nerve Agent Casualties," while the University of Maryland was paid more than $250,000 during the same decade for 3 contracts dealing with "Psychological Studies of the Effects of Chemical Warfare Agents."

While most colleges like the Universities of Maryland, Utah, and Washington received anywhere from 1 to 3 contracts over the 20-year testing period, the University of Pennsylvania's six contracts totaled $650,000, plus another $126,000 awarded to Kligman's private research lab, Ivy Research, for similar "threshold" drug studies.[17] The largest dollar value contract awarded to any institution was a $326,840 contract to the University of

Pennsylvania in March of 1964. Not only the size but also the nature of that contract was unprecedented. As the inspector general's report clearly stated:

> First, it was the first known contract that the Medical Research Laboratories entered into involving prison inmates. Second, it was the first indication found that the contract investigators may not have been fully prepared to conduct experiments with humans at the outset of the program. Finally, the records of the execution of that contract indicated that one of the purposes of the contract was to allow military medical investigators to conduct experiments using prison inmates as their subjects.[18]

The report elaborated on what the Chemical Corps Medical Contract project officer found when he visited the Philadelphia prison in November 1964.

> Throughout the entire three-day period, testing was hampered by equipment, such as needles, syringes and alcohol sponges, not being readily available. On the second day of testing, no medical personnel other than ourselves, were present, nor did any appear, or make contact with us prior to our leaving Friday afternoon.

The project officer recommended:

> It is our opinion that in order for this program to be successful, there needs to be guidance and supervision of the testing by the contractors. This is especially important in this early stage of the program for training of the nursing personnel and establishing standard operating procedures.[19]

These criticisms, and their implications about the validity of various studies done at Holmesburg, are interesting when we consider that for ten years previous to this Army contract, the Holmesburg research unit had been conducting hundreds of medical experiments.

V

One Army medical officer who was present for those initial inmate experiments and was dismayed by the prison's general unpreparedness for such delicate scientific testing was James S. Ketchum, a psychiatrist with a long and impressive medical career. A graduate of Columbia College, Ketchum received his medical degree from Cornell

University Medical School and took additional psychiatric training at such institutions as the Letterman in San Francisco, Walter Reed Army Hospital in Washington, D.C., and Stanford University. He has held several important positions with the military such as chief of the Army's clinical research, behavioral science, and psychiatry divisions, and has taught psychiatry at Emory, Baylor, the University of Califonia at Los Angeles, and the University of Texas Medical School. He has also written numerous articles, reports, and book chapters on drug research and psychopharmacology.

At the time of the Holmesburg experiments, Dr. Ketchum was a ranking research psychopharmacologist stationed at Edgewood Arsenal, the Army's hub for chemical warfare studies. His early visits to Holmesburg were unsettling; the facility was not prepared to do sensitive and dangerous psychopharmacologic testing. Even though he was a junior officer and had considerably less medical experience than Albert Kligman, the program's director, he "chewed out" the senior physician for his lackadaisical preparation. "I overstepped my authority," recalls Ketchum in an interview.[20] "I was not pleased with the quality of work there. I was not satisfied with the way he was using our initial subjects and I expressed myself rather assertively." Ketchum instructed Kligman to "put up some trailers in the prison yard and to get some appropriate staff." Ketchum recalls that while Kligman promised to hire a psychopharmacologist, he never did. Ketchum thinks that request may have prompted the arrival of Dr. Herbert Copelan, Kligman's second in command at the prison, but adds: "I was not particularly impressed with his pharmacological skills. He had none."

Ketchum was not alone in expressing his dissatisfaction with overall testing conditions. Lieutenant Colonel M. G. Bottiglieri, another of Edgewood's clinical researchers, wrote Dr. Kligman a memo blasting the university program's psychological reports as "pure gibberish...absolutely useless...nothing but a list of clichés seemingly pasted together without consideration of coherence in an attempt to provide a facade of competence and ability."[21] He added, "It seems incredible that [a psychologist] with...apparent qualifications would attempt to palm off such shoddy and psychologically naive material in response to our request."

When told that inmates and civilian technicians considered Copelan a competent and business-like physician, Ketchum didn't doubt it. He says Copelan was a good internist, but the Army was interested in numerous, potentially mind-disabling pharmacological experiments. Experienced and properly trained staff needed to be on site. In addition, a suitable physical environment was critical. Because test subjects under the influence of experimental drugs could injure themselves or others, walls and floors required padding and all furniture had to be pliable, with hard edges and corners padded.

Dr. Ketchum believes that the Army's relationship with the university and Dr. Kligman emerged out of the search for a facility more suitable to large-scale drug studies than Edgewood. "We only had facilities for certain tests and the ability to test ten to a dozen different compounds. It was a logistical problem. Edgewood could house only a few test volunteers at a time."[22] Dr. Frederick Sidell, another Army physician involved in the chemical studies at Edgewood, said; "Holmesburg looked sophisticated and adequate for test purposes," and after "some minor problems" at its inception, the prison studies proved "very helpful to the Army."[23]

Dr. Ketchum's initial visits to Holmesburg as a technical adviser to the experiments rapidly led him to conclude that the Army "was more conscientious than the civilians were" about scientific study and safety.[24] Kligman was told in fairly blunt terms to upgrade his staff and equipment. "My personal standards were pretty high and I recommended certain things for the experiments to ensure their quality and professionalism." After 30 years, Ketchum is still amazed that Kligman, a dermatologist who was not qualified to oversee experiments using mind-altering drugs, never hired a psychopharmacologist to direct the tests. Interestingly, the importance of the proper testing personnel was not completely lost on Kligman. According to Alan Katz, the licensed pharmacist who worked for the University of Pennsylvania research program at Holmesburg for 10 years, Kligman asked Katz "to sign a document for the Army....He believed my signature gave weight and credence to [the application for] a government license."[25] Katz repeatedly makes clear, however, that he did not claim to have the expertise of a pharmachologist and the he "never, ever, became involved in the Army experiments. McBride and Copelan ran that operation. I had nothing to do with it." Katz's firm, almost self-protective, denial of any involvement in the Army experiments is not unique. According to a number of Dr. Kligman's former students and research employees, the threat of public exposure and the fear of lawsuits continues to haunt them decades later.[26]

Others, such as Ketchum, find this view overblown. The experiments, he claims, were generally harmless and well monitored. He says: "The Holmesburg inmates rated pretty much the same as the Army subjects. Overall the survey was useful. Speedier results...helped us confirm earlier findings...and one signal achievement—Physostigmine."[27] This drug, which had been considered useful for postoperative sluggishness of the intestines, proved a very effective antidote to several deliriants, such as atropine and scopolamine, administered in the tests.

The reactions of the prisoners who received these drugs, whether by injection, orally, or aerosol mist, varied considerably. Some acted out in potentially dangerous ways, like Johnnie Williams, while others slept through the experiment. Dr. Ketchum recalls that while Johnnie Williams was dislodging the toilet, cell door, and generally scaring the hell out of all in attendance, "the guy in the cell next to him was lying there blissful, saying he was on a heroin high. There was quite a range of subjective responses to the drug." Because of the varied reactions, especially the terrifying hallucinations of "giant ants and spiders coming out of the walls," most inmates who went through the trailer experiments believe they were part of secret LSD tests. Chemicals such as atropine, scopolamine, and BZ were unknown to the inmates, but LSD had become part of both the mainstream and criminal lexicon.

Many of the inmates had been heavy drug users, but the vast majority had limited their use to alcohol, marijuana, and heroin. LSD would never become the popular drug among inner-city criminals that it became among the more affluent and college-educated counterculture. Even with an inmate experienced with LSD, according to Dr. Ketchum, the varied drug "reactions could be easily confused by both doctors and laymen. Only experienced pharmacologists could discern the difference." Ketchum explains that the stimulant LSD could create very "inventive and fantastic images." Anticholinergics such as atropine, on the other hand, were "depressants that block neuro-transmitters and obliterate the ability to evaluate what goes on in our heads." He says it was very common for an individual injected with scopolamine or BZ to have fantastic visions of "animals, mice, and bugs." By 1966, according to Ketchum, the army had lost interest in LSD as an incapacitant, and LSD tests ended.

Ketchum says that much of the reason volunteers were kept uninformed arose out of the perceived need for government "security." On the subject of informed consent, Ketchum regrets the cursory nature of the briefings, but defends the Army's concern and fear of stolen secrets. He says he occasionally briefed the inmates himself.

> I told them we had a drug we want to test and it has been tested on animals and soldiers, and it does have some effect on your capacity to do certain functions [problems] and if things get rough, we have proper antidotes....We did not tell them the name of the compound because we wanted to avoid bias in testing...and maintain secrecy....If some of the subjects did get delirious on the tests and had higher reactions than we expected, we backed off, because we were not prepared for serious reactions. All of our intensive studies were done at the hospital at Edgewood; not in a prison.[28]

Ketchum says the "threat of chemical warfare" was very real during the Cold War, and the Army's research had the full support of President Kennedy's administration. There was great "fear of the Russians and their interest in LSD. It was a jittery period—the space race and the nuclear build-up." It was of major importance, he says, "to keep the Soviets from discovering what we [were] doing." The incapacitants we were working on "would have had great appeal to them. We wanted to stay one step ahead."

As the years have passed, Ketchum has grown more disturbed with the "slanted picture that has been presented" about Edgewood's chemical experiments. He says the Army researchers have been portrayed by writers and film documentarians as "bad guys acting under a cloak of secrecy," but says that is not an accurate picture. He labels some of these individuals "victimologists" who are hoping to become "liberators of the truth," illuminating ill-conceived and haphazardly run LSD experiments on unwitting citizens. "Someone has got to try and bring up the truth," says Ketchum; he believes the Edgewood studies were prudently handled and necessary for national security. "I am not saying every study was defensible, but ours were pretty legitimate and professional."

Dr. Ketchum repeatedly emphasizes the critical importance of the inmates to scientific advancement, and the precautionary measures observed to ensure their safety. He gives several examples to demonstrate the Army's professionalism and concern. In a test of the potent substance EA 3167, the testers received "startling results" after a "40 percent increase" in the dosage. The doctor stresses that "we immediately stopped our testing when the men showed dramatic changes. We were just interested in the threshold dose." On another occasion, a junior officer sent to Holmesburg to observe an experiment returned to Maryland and nonchalantly reported that the tests had gone well, but a couple of the test subjects had still been reeling when he left the penal facility. "'What are you doing here?'" replied Ketchum, alarmed. "'You should be up there.' As soon as he told me what he had seen, I told him to get his stuff; 'You're going back up there.' We went back on a Friday night and spent the weekend observing and caring for the men." Ketchum says he and the Army took the tests very seriously and that the "nature of the drugs caused concern. I went up there four or five times and stayed a couple of days each time."

There were some psychotropic experiments, however, about which Ketchum was unaware. According to Herbert Copelan's synopsis of a May 1970 experiment conducted by Ivy Research (Kligman's private lab) at Holmesburg, a test was "terminated prematurely because of syncopal reaction [sudden loss of consciousness] precipitated by retching after I.V. injection of Agent 926." The report stated that at

> 9:57 A.M. on 22 May 1970,...a 35-year-old white man, 6 feet 3 inches tall and 207.5 pounds, received an intravenous 113.2 ug. dose of Agent 926. About 30 seconds after injection, he reported nausea and slumped forward. He was immediately rolled back on the bed and his legs were elevated. He was ashen, unconscious and

motionless. His skin was not moist. No radial, precordial or cervical pulsation was seen or felt. About one minute after injection, or 15 seconds after being placed in the supine position without response, two or three precordial blows were given and regular sternal compression was started. Mouth to nose ventilation was begun some 30 seconds after the start of sternal compression.[29]

Fortunately, the patient responded to these efforts and showed a normal electrocardiogram and blood pressure reading 2 hours after the injection, although he remained nauseated and bed ridden. The other 19 subjects recovered as well.

Dr. Ketchum recalls EA 926 well. He says, "The drug defied category. It was very potent in animals because of its knockdown effect, [but] it was hard to know what effect it would have in man." Described as a member of the "morphine or pain killer category," EA 926 was feared to be in the Soviet drug arsenal and a threat to U.S. personnel. Ketchum says he and his Army colleagues had a lot of misgivings about the drug and decided not to test it. "We agonized over it at Edgewood. The drug had great appeal but it was rejected as unsafe." When informed that it had been given to Philadelphia prison inmates, the Army doctor replied: "If it was, I was not part of it." But the CIA probably was. The testing of drugs like EA 926 and EA 3167 was part of a drug testing program begun in the mid-1960s and code-named Project OFTEN.

VI

Since the end of World War II, the CIA had been preoccupied with the potential benefit and threat of truth serums and exotic drugs. Whereas the Army investigated drugs that incapacitated, the CIA pursued drugs that could control the mind. During the Korean War, two secret programs, code-named ULTRA and NAOMI, were established "to investigate whether and how it was possible to modify an individual's behavior by covert means."[30] Everything from hallucinogenic mushrooms to BZ was studied by CIA investigators. In the attempt to create the perfect CIA operative, brainwashing, hypnosis, electroshock, personality assessments, and a host of other techniques were added to the drug list. The prospect of programming an individual to do one's bidding—a human magic bullet more dependable than traditional agents—was overpowering. Most, if not all, of these initiatives proved useless; the vision of a simple, one-step drug to facilitate everything from police investigations to the unmasking of foreign spies was considerably more difficult to realize than the agency had expected.

Much of the documentation concerning the CIA's role in human experimentation was destroyed in 1973 under the orders of Richard Helms, the agency's director. President Richard Nixon's decision to remove Helms and name a new director spurred Helms to order the destruction of embarrassing files, particularly those dealing with human experimentation. Furthermore, some CIA initiatives were considered too controversial for written transcription. "Closely guarded" experiments had their results "conveyed verbally," leading to "sparse documentation" of the projects.[31] Stansfield Turner, then chief of the CIA, told inquiring senators at one high-profile hearing that it had been agency policy "to maintain no records of the planning and approval of test programs" during much of their human research work.[32]

The CIA's early investigations centered on the possibilities of dlysergic acid diethylamide, LSD. Discovered by accident in 1943 by Dr. Albert Hoffmann, a Swiss chemist working for the Sandoz Pharmaceutical firm, LSD was several times more potent than other mind-altering drugs like mescaline. In an attempt to discover how and why LSD worked as it did, and what antidotes could be used against it, the CIA sank hundreds of thousands of dollars into a whole new field of research. Funneled through front groups such as the Josiah Macy, Jr., Foundation and the Geschickter Fund for Medical Research, the agency was able to pay significant monetary stipends to worthy institutions willing to investigate new drugs.[33]

By the mid-1960s, the agency was ready to further explore "ways for predictably influencing human behavior through the use of drugs."[34] In early 1966, it established a "behavioral pharmacology program" in order to develop the "capability to manipulate human behavior in a predictable manner through the use of drugs and to devise defensive means...to protect agency personnel from drugs clandestinely administered by the opposition." Such drugs would also be useful in "interrogation situations, penetration of guarded areas, covert action, and paramilitary operations."

Part of this new effort, code-named Project OFTEN, was designed to test in animals a wide assortment of "drugs and chemical compounds having desired behavioral effects" that could then be "clinically evaluated with human subjects." (One of OFTEN's goals was to "come up with a compound that could stimulate a heart attack or a stroke in the targeted individual, or perhaps a new hallucinogen to cause the targeted individual to act bizarrely."[35]) The human experiments were done jointly with the U.S. Army at the Chemical Research and Development Laboratory at Edgewood Arsenal, chosen because of their existing foreign drug work, their experience with EA 3167, and their program of using human volunteers. The CIA, aware of the U.S. Army's varied experiments with chemical warfare agents at Holmesburg, saw the same advantages the Army had in a continuous population confined under controlled conditions. And from the CIA's more cynical point of view, prisoners offered further advantages: they were for the most part uneducated, isolated, had few substantive ties to their communities that would make inquiries, and they were financially destitute enough to make them willing to take risks in exchange for payment.[36]

According to a 1969 CIA memorandum, early accounts of Project OFTEN's progress were positive; attempts to "identify pharmacological agents with new and unusual effects" were showing "interesting properties" and potential.[37] One report disclosed that "fifty newly synthesized, novel compounds" had been screened, and exhibited "promising behavioral activity."[38] More than 400 compounds had been acquired with the expectation of analyzing a minimum of 50 per year. The candidate compounds were tested on mice, rats, cats, and monkeys with the goal of establishing which agents best induced rage, lethargy, disorientation, and incapacitation. "Based on early findings," the project was expected to have a "major impact on the agency's potential for controlling human performance and for defense against exploitation of key, national personnel by hostile intelligence services."[39] By 1971, annual drug screenings had risen to 120 annually but a "back-log of over 26,000 compounds" still existed.[40]

It was apparently this last point that brought Holmesburg prisoners into the CIA's drug research. It was deemed "essential" that the drug research program be carried forward and "countermeasures" to the threat of Soviet activity in pharmacology be implemented as soon as possible. Interestingly, although the CIA's advisory panel, consisting of members from the Office of Research and Development and the Technical Services Division, agreed that a "rapid response" was necessary, there was a "serious split" over how to proceed. The conflict focused on "the testing with human subjects of drugs significantly affecting human behavior, but rejected for clinical use." Evidently, some panel members were dismayed about the "political sensitivity" and the "unpredictable long-range clinical effects" of the drugs to be tested. The majority, however, believed the "risks" had been "minimized" and that the work on "psychopharmacological incapacitating and behavior control agents" should go forward agressively.[41]

The records show that the Army doctors at Edgewood were retained by the CIA in 1971. One drug that particularly interested the CIA and that Holmesburg prisoners had previously tested for the Army was EA 3167, believed to be the centerpeice of Soviet behavior control studies. As Dr. Ketchum's confidential 1973 report states, "EA 3167 is a highly potent, extremely long-lasting glycolate belladonoid with a steep dose-response curve" that is capable of leaving the subject "delirious for a period of 1 to 14 days."[42] It was the high potency of EA 3167 that the CIA found so attractive.

A summary of Project OFTEN, developed for the agency's director of research and development and labeled "secret," stated that $37,000 was transferred to Edgewood on February 17, 1971, "to extend the Army's research on EA 3167" and "include the oral and trans-dermal routes" since these posed the greatest "potential threats to U.S. VIPs and other key personnel."[43] (Interestingly, neither Dr. Ketchum nor Dr. Sidell knew about the CIA investigations of EA 3167 at Edgewood and Holmesburg. Dr. Sidell says the only occasion he knew of linking the CIA and EA 3167 was in the early 1970s when "former CIA workers loyal to President Nixon, tried to put EA 3167 on the steering wheel of Jack Anderson's car to make him a little bonkers. They assumed it would be passed through the skin although our work had always been through injection."[44]) Once more, Holmesburg prisoners were used in the tests.

Agency documents disclose that testing of EA 3167 was terminated in January 1973. In 1979 Stansfield Turner admitted to Congress: "No such magic brew as the popular notion of truth serum exists."[45] The then–CIA chief said, "Even under the best conditions," drugs "will elicit an output contaminated by deception, fantasy, [and] garbled speech." In addition, Turner said, "both normal individuals and psychopaths" can learn "to resist drug interrogation." In fact, this ability to withstand drugs was best exemplified in "well-adjusted individuals with good defenses and good emotional control."

For several years thereafter, the CIA grappled with difficulties caused by the haphazard record keeping of their covert human drug experiments. A search was made for clear and accurate documentation of the Agency's role not only to appease alarmed legislators and public citizens, but also to ensure "medical follow-up" for those "persons who may suffer adverse effects from participation" in the drug experiments.[46] In short, EA 3167 was considered so potent and long-lasting that the test subjects had to be located and examined "without regard to who may have sponsored the tests."

There is no written record, however, to show that follow-up contacts were made, and conversations with key Edgewood personnel disclose no attempts by the CIA, or other government personnel, to track down former EA 3167 test subjects. Apparently, government bureaucrats gave up in defeat when Dr. Kligman told investigators he had destroyed all his old files along with the lists naming the experimental subjects. But if they had dug a little deeper, they would have found the cell block log books that charted the passage of prisoners on and off individual cell blocks to and from the hubs of experimental activity, H Block and the Army trailers. The 1968–69 H Block Log Book, for example, discloses numerous references to the "U of P Army Study in the Trailers," next to the names of Holmesburg inmates.[47] These were the prisoners who participated in the Army experiments and were confined in the trailers for the duration of their tests. On July 21, 1968, for example as indicated in the log book, inmates Bruce Agnew (I-1640) and James Walker (I-8388) were "received" on H Block to take part in the "U of P Army Study." Two days later on July 23, Agnew was "transferred" to J Block and Walker was "transferred" to A Block when they "completed the Army

Study." In many cases such "Army Study" notations were highlighted in red ink to draw attention to an inmate's participation in special activities. The H Block Log Book covering the period from April 30, 1968, to May 7, 1969, discloses the names of 95 inmates who spent time in the Army trailers, names available for follow-up contact by the government investigators. Moreover, the Army's own files, compiled from the periodic reports of Drs. Kligman and Copelan, include many names of test subjects. Through the Holmesburg log books and the Army test records, it would have been relatively easy to confirm who received EA 3167, EA 926, or any of the potent psychotropic drugs tested on the prisoners, and to conduct a medical follow-up.

VII

In the mid-1960s, Dr. Kligman devoted "three years of continuous research to the nature of the hardening process" of skin for the U.S. Army.[48] According to a May 1967 annual report from Drs. Kligman and Copelan to the Edgewood Arsenal's Medical Research Laboratories, "three types of irritant exposure" were examined: "(1) occlusive patch tests under an impermeable dressing, (2) surface painting without a cover and (3) arm and hand immersion." Substances that were used in patch tests on the backs of prisoners included a long list of abrasive and toxic chemicals: "phenol, salicylic acid, coal tar, octylamine, cationic detergents (Hyamines), anionic detergents (sodium lauryl sulfate and soaps), fatty acids, (caproic and propionic) hydrochloric acid, sodium hydroxide, croton oil, zinc chloride, benzene, ethylene glycol monomethyl ether, hexane, DM50, and mercuric chloride."[49]

Tests showed that "some degree of hardening is obtainable with all of these substances." Some, however, were so dangerous that their contact with human skin precluded hardening. Hydrochloric acid and sodium hydroxide, for instance, were such "destructive chemicals" that when applied they induced intense inflammation and "no real hardening [was] achievable."

For other substances, the prison doctor determined that the "length of daily exposure proved exceedingly important" to hardening. It was, for example, "generally impossible" to produce hardening if patches were worn continuously. Patches "applied [for] 24 hours every third day" hardened the skin, "but [took] a longer time." The most successful technique, the experimenters discovered, was "one to four hour exposures on a daily basis, using chemical concentrations which produced a maximum inflammatory reaction in about 10 to 14 days....Accommodation," as the report's authors referred to it, was "usually achieved in six to eight weeks."

Surprisingly, the surface application experiments were "mainly tried on the forehead." Kligman and Copelan were "interest[ed] in acnes," and discovered that "the face turns out to be quite satisfactory; it inflames quickly and hardens rather swiftly."

The best results were obtained with 15 percent croton oil in equal parts of acetone and ethylene glycol monomethyl ether, 10 percent phenol in water and 30 percent zinc chloride. With these, a severe inflammatory reaction is provoked which reaches a peak in about 10 days, accompanied by a rather frightening amount of crusting. This separates and healing ensues in about six weeks at which time the skin is clinically normal except for pigmentation.

Dr. Kligman was quite proud of his work in this area and told the Army the "promising" results were "being pursued vigorously."[50] As we have seen, the prisoners were less enthusiastic about the cavalier approach to scarring chemicals applied to their faces.

In an article coauthored by Kligman and published in the *Journal of Investigative Dermatology* in 1967, the arm and hand immersion experiments revealed that the best hardening agents proved to be sodium lauryl sulfate (SLS) and sodium tetrachloro-phenol. The article said some chemicals proved to be "severely limiting" because of their "systemic toxicity."[51] When they used pure, undiluted ethylene glycol monomethyl ether, "three of the test subjects exhibited psychotic reactions (hallucinations, stupor, etc.) within two weeks and had to be hospitalized." Pure, undiluted dimethyl-acetamide worked even faster, but "headaches and febrile reactions" ended the test. After several years of these chemical experiments on the skin, Kligman arrived at the "inescapable conclusion" that solid hardening "is attainable only if the skin passes through a very intense inflammatory phase with swelling, redness, scaling, and crusting." It is difficult to establish how many scores of city prisoners underwent these uncomfortable, and sometimes painful, skin experiments. Kligman and Copelan said the skins of a dozen inmates had been kept hardened for a year on just SLS and chlorinated phenol. These men would more than likely display discolored skin permanently, for "the first layer never quite returns to normal; its cells tend to be more swollen and it thereby has a translucent appearance." An additional finding concerning racial differences disclosed that "there can be no question that the Negro is more resistant to irritation." Generally, the authors said, "higher concentrations" of chemicals "are required to obtain peak dermatitis."

Some experiments united the inmates against the scientists. When allergens such as nickel and neomycin were introduced into the experiment, the "project turned out to be unfeasible." Inflammation lasted for weeks without the skin becoming hard. The willingness of the subjects to continue "diminished to zero...and the study was terminated."[52]

When I asked Dr. Ketchum about the usefulness and scope of these skin-hardening experiments, he replied that he had not been aware of them, but that the search for a protective coating of hardened skin was important to the military. Soldiers were exposed to all sorts of foreign and deadly elements while in open field combat, and the discovery of chemical compounds that protected the men's skin would have provided a tremendous defensive advantage. Rather than armor made from iron, the skin itself would be armor.

Although many inmates participated in experiments similar in design to the skin-hardening studies, none interviewed knew if they had been part of the Army tests. In fact, none of those interviewed was told of the Army's association with such tests, and because the tests were held on H Block and not in the Army trailers, the subjects were under the impression that the hand and arm immersion tests were relatively harmless "soap studies."

VIII

When Kligman informed the Army that the "trailers were installed and placed in full operation," it signaled a new and frightening chapter in the dermatologist's experimental portfolio, one that he was not medically trained to pursue.[53] Located between H and G Blocks, each

trailer was expected to "accommodate eight subjects for periods ranging from several hours to several weeks." Kligman informed the Army
that the trailers had increased the efficiency of his operation "significantly," allowing "twenty-four subjects per month" to be tested,
although more could be handled when "special need arises."

The skin-hardening experiments may have caused their fair share of
physical and emotional distress, but it was the trailers—and the evident effects of mind-disabling drugs experiments that occurred within
them—that really became the hallmark of the Kligman/University of
Pennsylvania human research program. An examination of the monthly
and annual reports Kligman sent the Army illuminates much about the
once-secret program, from volunteer payscales and program goals to staff
additions and test results. The corrrespondence verifies Dr. Ketchum's
recollection that the Army repeatedly pressed Kligman to hire suitable
staff, and that Kligman agreed to hire a "neuro-pharmacologist," but no
such hiring was reported.[54] Kligman did inform the Army that because
of "the prolonged effects of some of the experimental chemicals, and
the duration involved for continual clinical research, the present
inmate-subject pay scale has been revised." He also reported that "a
subject used in the study of a parasympatholytic agent...attempted to
do bodily harm to his cell partner," and that some inmates who had
been involved in psychotropic testing were "unexpectedly dis-
charged." But, he assured the Army, "several attempts to contact [the
former inmate] at his home" had been made.

The annual report for the year ending March 31, 1966, catalogs
details of the program: the review of more than 3,000 inmate jack-
ets; the rejection of 2,600 inmates; the subsequent physical and
mental screening; and the 322 MMPIs that were administered and
resulted in another 95 subjects rejected.[55] This screening led to the
selection of 148 inmates for experimentation, and the report provides information on the chemical agents (or their Army codes)
being tested alongside the number of inmates involved.

Agent	Number of Subjects
1-G	16
1-J	10
CAR 302,196	41

CAR 302,368	20
Scopolamine	8
Atropine	25
EA 3167	12
GA 3520	8
Ditran	8

In the mid- and late 1960s, these drugs, plus numerous variations, became the focus of the Army's Medical Research Division. From 1964 to 1973, Holmesburg prisoners were subjected to an assortment of these mind-disabling chemicals. Examples of the agents and their impact on the test subjects as described in Kligman's and Copelan's various reports follow.

Agent 282. A glycolate class chemical. Inmates described their reactions as "groggy," "light-headed," "woozy," "top heavy," and "drugged." Some claimed they had "watery eyes" or were "cross-eyed" with "double vision." Two subjects said the walls of the room seemed to be moving or floating "like the sides of a tent blowing in the wind." A few subjects hallucinated, "seeing faces or insects and one...had auditory hallucinations [heard music]."[56]

Agent 834. "Subjects reported they felt 'high', 'dazed', or 'light-headed'...unsteady...on first standing up....Subjects swayed while standing and walking, sometimes brushing against the walls....Heaviness of the eyes,....'seeing double', [and]...significant mental impairment." The inmates also suffered "hallucinations," such as "crawling ants" and other forms of insect and animal life.[57]

CAR 302,212. Subjects suffered from "'lightheadedness', or mild 'dizziness.'...Inmates became drowsy and...fell asleep,...swayed on standing,...brushing against walls" as they tried to walk. They demonstrated "slight impairment of thinking" and "at higher doses...blurring of near vision."[58]

CAR 302,368. An intermediate-acting drug similar to scopolamine. Inmates suffered from "lightheadedness," "feeling high," and "unsteadiness," their "legs felt rubbery," and their "speech...became slurred." They said the "walls and ceilings drifted away...thinking slowed [and] drowsiness appeared. The subjects felt they lacked drive."[59]

Agent 1-11 (atropine sulfate). "Consciousness during the test appeared dull. Several subjects had symptoms suggesting mild delirium. They reported dreams that were primarily visual and in color....The hallucinations occasionally were frightening. Subjects had difficulty distinguishing reality from fantasy....A few subjects complained of minor symptoms for periods as long as six weeks after receiving the agent."[60]

Agent 668. "Heaviness of the eyes and unsteadiness were the dominant central symptoms....They felt mildly high or intoxicated....Subjects were slightly drowsy, dozed more and daydreamed a little more than normal....A few visual illusions and...hallucinations were reported. Occasionally cracks or spots were interpreted as insects or faces....A few subjects reported apparent motion of the walls after one or two hours. The walls seemed to be breathing."[61]

IX

Holmesburg prisoners tested more than a dozen highly potent mind-altering drugs during the nearly ten-year relationship between the Army and the county prison in Philadelphia. Hundreds of incarcerated men, willing to risk their physical and mental health for payment, were unwittingly injected with some of the most potent chemicals the U.S. military and the CIA had in their arsenals. Though the Army's physicians felt the Holmesburg Prison experiments were "very helpful" in pursuing their scientific goals, most likely only a few of the test subjects would agree.

For Johnnie Williams, the aging warrior of Philadelphia's streets and violent prison cell blocks, the mental and physical wounds remain. Moreover, he no longer sees doctors as helpful, respected pillars of society. Williams was recently hit by a car and he reports that the hospital personnel were "concerned about hip, leg, and back injuries."[62] But Williams refused treatment and limped out of the emergency ward. "I'm paranoid about doctors. I'm scared of 'em," he says. "I don't want anything to do with doctors or hospitals. I'm afraid of 'em."

Five

"I Am Not Part of the Program."

I

On August 26, 1963, the Division of Licensing and Regulation of the U.S. Atomic Energy Commission (AEC) received an application from Dr. Albert M. Kligman for a By-Product Material License, a document that would allow him to work with radioactive isotopes.[1] Like a number of his medical colleagues around the country during the Cold War, Kligman had become intrigued by the possibilities of radioactive medicine. Once again, he used Holmesburg prisoners in his scientific expedition.

Although the postwar attraction of nuclear medicine was powerful, only a small, select vanguard in the medical community performed experiments using radioactive material on prison inmates. But while the experiments were few in number, they ranged from fairly innocuous to quite dangerous. Prisoners in Utah were administered radioactive isotopes and some had blood "removed, irradiated and returned" to their bodies.[2] "They told us nothing about the tests," said one prison volunteer. "They just said it wouldn't bother us."[3]

In the early 1960s, inmates at Colorado State Penitentiary were part of an "experiment designed to determine the survival time and characteristics of red blood cells during periods of rapid red cell formation and severe iron deficiency."[4] The studies used radioactive iron and phosphorus as tagging mechanisms. Similar experimental initiatives were carried out at Oklahoma State Penitentiary (routine metabolic studies of experimental drugs using tracer amounts of radionuclides), at Stateville Prison in Illinois (measurements of radium burden received from drinking water), and at California's San Quentin Prison (tracking the movement of iron from plasma to red blood cells using a radioactive marker).[5]

II

The best-known and most fully researched examples of prisoner irradiation are the twin cases of Oregon and Washington. They ran from 1963 to 1973 under the sponsorship of the AEC. These experiments, which were designed to measure the effects of radiation on the male reproductive system and sperm cell development, grew out of a concern about radiation hazards to astronauts in the nascent space program, as well as workers in nuclear power and weapons plants. The experiments were directed by Dr. Carl G. Heller, a preeminent researcher and the leading endocrinologist of his day, and Dr. Heller's protege, Dr. C. Alvin Paulsen.[6]

In the Oregon case, Dr. Heller designed a study "to test the effects of radiation on the somatic and germinal cells of the testes, the doses of radiation that would produce changes or induce damage in spermatogenic cells, the amount of time it would take for cell production to recover, and the effects of radiation on hormone excretion."[7] In the experiment, a test subject sat with his scrotum in a small plastic box filled with warm water; the box was bracketed by sets of X-ray tubes for uniform irradiation. Every subject was required to get a vasectomy—usually at the conclusion of the study—in order to ensure that chromosomal damage would not lead to "fathering genetically damaged children."[8] During the decade that Dr. Heller conducted his study, he received government grants totaling $1.1 million.[9]

A test subject was paid $5 a month, $10 for each testicular biopsy (usually five or more), plus $100 when he was vasectomized at the end of the program; subjects endured skin burns, pain from biopsies, testicular inflammation, and bleeding into the scrotum from the biopsies. Interestingly, the Roman Catholic Church prohibited Catholics from participating in the experiment, not because the tests were dangerous, but because the church objected to its members masturbating to provide semen samples. By 1973, after 67 inmates had been irradiated, the "rapidly changing research ethics environment" caused the termination of the Oregon experiment.[10] Three years later a number of test subjects filed lawsuits alleging poorly supervised research and lack of informed consent. In 1979 the suits were settled out of court. Nine prisoners shared $2,215 in damages.

The AEC selected Dr. Paulsen to initiate a half-million-dollar research program in 1963 after several workers at the Hanford nuclear plant in Washington state were accidentally exposed to radiation. Paulsen said his goal was to establish a "reasonably safe dose of ionizing radiation to the testes,...[to discover] what dose would cause some change in sperm production and...to determine the scenario of recovery."[11] Dr. Paulsen decided to use a standard General Electric X-ray machine instead of Heller's custom model, and to advertise for volunteers on the prison's bulletin board. Notices such as the following informed inmates of the experiment:

> Subject: Additional Volunteers for Radiation Research Project. The project concerns effects of radiation on human testicular function and the results of the project will be utilized in the safety of personnel working around atomic steam plants, etc....It is possible that those men receiving the higher dosages may be temporarily, or even permanently, sterilized. It should be understood that when sterilized in this manner, a man still has the same desires and can still perform as he always has....Submit to surgical biopsy. (This is a simple procedure performed under local anesthesia. It is not a very painful procedure.)[12]

Paulsen's program was terminated in 1970 after questions arose over the issues of informed consent, the nontherapeutic nature of the studies, and legal liability.[13]

Years after their participation in these dangerous experiments, many former prisoners remain angry about how their ignorance and lack of sophistication were used against them. "We can be blamed for being duped," said Robert Garrison in a 1994 newpaper interview.[14] "[N]obody ever sat us down and explained what the tests were all about and what the complications were." Garrison said, "I can't even get a doctor to diagnose my problems, let alone give me treatment for them. I shouldn't have to scream to get some kind of results. I'm a human being too." Phillip King took part in the Oregon tests in 1969 and still complains of groin pain so severe that it prevents him from sitting down. "I took part in the tests and now I'm in a lot of pain," says King, who struggles to make ends meet doing odd jobs in Portland. "I don't know what I'm owed, but I think I'm owed something."[15] Harold Bibeau, another former Oregon State Prison test subject, was exposed to 18 rads' (doses of radiation); "an average modern X-ray ranges between 0.1 and 1 rad." He has recently discovered lumps on his thigh and back. When asked why he subjected himself to experimentation, the former soldier claims that it was a chance to perform a patriotic duty. "I was just told that it was a way to serve my country even though I was in prison....And I bought it."[16]

III

Until he established his lab in Holmesburg Prison, Albert Kligman's experience with radioactivity was limited to the comparatively simple X-ray machines that were common diagnostic tools by mid-century. To Kligman and other dermatologists, X-rays were a key weapon in the fight against ringworm. In a 1954 coauthored article reporting on a study supported by a grant from the U.S. Public Health Service, he wrote: "The depilatory effect of superficial X-rays is curative in almost all cases of epidemic tinea capitis [ringworm] due to Microsporum audouini."[17] Since the head is a spheroid that does not lend itself to uniform irradiation, Kligman used the Adamson-Kienbock method in which radiation was "delivered over five unshielded focal points which are approximately five inches apart." Because "certain radiologists [were] sufficiently fearful of the potential damage" from this procedure, particularly about "the quantities of radiation absorbed in the...overlapping...areas," Kligman looked at the effects of this radiation method on children (some possibly as young as 2 or 3 years old).[18] He concluded from his clinical data that "the Adamson-Kienbock technique is quite safe for the routine epilation of fungus-infected scalps, provided that it is done by experienced personnel with well-calibrated equipment."[19] Although some dermatologists still were not prepared to call the procedure completely successful—because the patient's hair never grew back—X-ray epilation was routinely administered to destroy the highly contagious fungi.[20] Dr. Kligman continued to experiment with X-ray therapy on various other skin diseases.

Nearly a decade later in 1963, the same year as Heller's and Paulsen's prison experiments on the West Coast, Kligman sought a license from the AEC to conduct new inquiries into radioactive medicine. According to the application, Dr. Kligman planned to perform "physiological and pharmacological studies on the absorption of materials through the skin by topical application, intradermal injection and by iontophoresis."[21] The application may have confused the AEC about who the authorized users were who were trained and qualified to handle radioactive materials at Holmesburg Prison.

Kligman's application specified the radioactive isotopes he intended to use. They included Carbon[14], Mercury[203], Nickel[63], Arsenic[74], Zirconium[95], Sulfur[35], Iodine[131], and Hydrogen[3]; the application also catalogued the technical instruments, the operating procedures, and the members of the critically important Isotope Safety Committee who would supervise the procedures. The radiation protection officer was the centerpiece of this committee, and it was his job to "insure proper storage...of radioactive materials....inspect periodically, without advance notice, the operating conditions in all laboratories where work with radioisotopes is in progress...[and] call attention to any infractions of rules and regulations."[22] In short, "the entire program involving the use of labelled materials in humans" would be under his supervision. The application identified the radiation protection officer as Dr. Benjamin Calesnick.

When interviewed and asked about his critical role in the Holmesburg experiments, Dr. Calesnick grew agitated. "That's not correct," he replied firmly. "I did not operate radioactive material testing at Holmesburg."[23] Professor Emeritus of Human Pharmacology at Hahnemann Medical College and Hospital in Philadelphia, Dr. Calesnick says he had no involvement whatsoever with the University of Pennsylvania's human experimentation program at the prison. When Dr. Calesnick inspected the 32-year-old AEC document, obtained through the Freedom of Information Act, he said: "[Kligman] was operating nuclear chemicals without the proper credentials or training. The whole damn thing was a fraud." He says that he has never entered Holmeburg, has never seen the protocol and application for the license, and had no association with the experiment.

As Calesnick recalls the history, "Hahnemann [Hospital] was a forerunner in the use of isotopes" and Kligman "had to get clearance for the acquisition and use [of radioactive materials]." Calesnick and Beatrice Troyan (Kligman's first wife) had been "classmates" and she "asked me to do a favor for him." Shortly thereafter, he received a "phone call" from Kligman. "He said, 'You got to help me out Ben.'" Apparently, Kligman needed a consultant on radioactive materials for upcoming experiments at Holmesburg. "I said, 'Sure Al.'" They hung up and Calesnick waited to be contacted about the details and scope of Kligman's application to the AEC. But Calesnick claims he "never had any [further] discussion" with Kligman about his project, and is equally adamant that he "never signed those applications" for AEC approval.

Not surprisingly, Dr. Calesnick thumbed through the AEC papers with great interest. His anger was obvious. Each time he saw his name mentioned in association with the Holmesburg project he grew more agitated. He remembers that he was contacted by the AEC informing him of a "problem at Holmesburg....I got a call from the AEC....[Kligman] was a sloppy worker and didn't have proper storage of the materials at the prison." Calesnick was distressed by the implications of the phone call; it indicated a perceived connection and responsibility for an experimentation program in which he had no role; he recalls asking for copies of the application "to check signatures....But they [the AEC] never sent it."

As Calesnick examined the old application and noted the list of radioactive materials presumably to be used on prisoners, he remarked "[Kligman] was trained to put ointments on skin,...what the hell was he doing with all this stuff?" Calesnick says Kligman always had a "reputation as an operator," as a man who knew "how to make money out of medicine." Human experimentation had become one of the fastest-growing and most financially rewarding fields in medicine, but you "needed big numbers" to secure corporate contracts and government grants. Echoing the comments of other physician-scientists, Calesnick says that because of a prison's

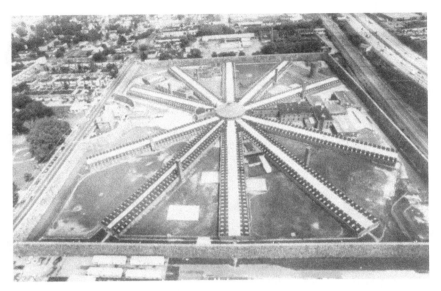

Constructed in 1896, Holmesburg Prison is typical of large, fortress-like penal institutions built in the 19th-century that incorporated spoke and wheel architecture. One of the three original U.S. Army trailers can be seen between H and G cellblocks (bottom, center). (© Urban Archives, Temple University, Philadelphia, PA)

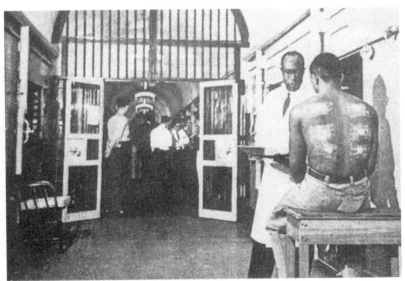

Solomon McBride, medical administrator of Holmesburg's human research, questions a test subject in H Block in February of 1966. (© Urban Archives, Temple University, Philadelphia, PA)

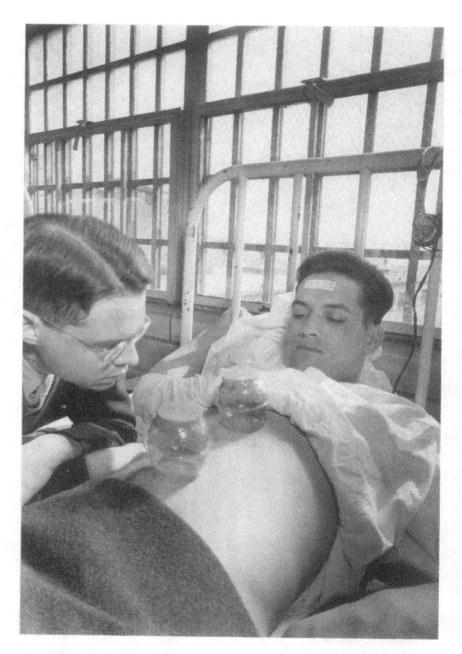

Malaria had a devastating impact on U.S. soldiers in the South Pacific. Over 400 prisoners volunteered at Stateville Penitentiary in Illinois during World War II to help find a cure for the tropical disease. Disease-carrying mosquitoes are shown biting the stomach of an inmate volunteer. (Myron Davis, *Life Magazine* © Time, Inc.)

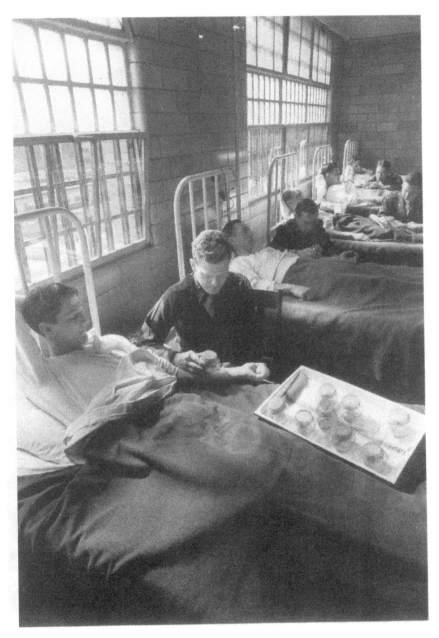

One of four prisons to host malaria studies, prisoners had to contend with high fevers, nausea, numerous experimental drugs, and periodic relapses. (Myron Davis, *Life Magazine* © Time, Inc.)

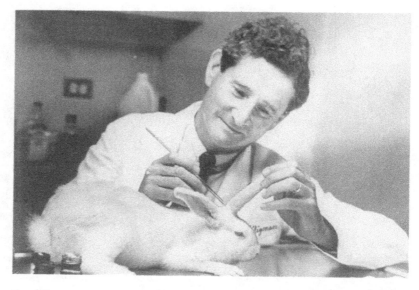

Dr. Albert Kligman conducts an experiment on a rabbit's ear in 1967.
(© Urban Archives, Temple University, Philadelphia, PA)

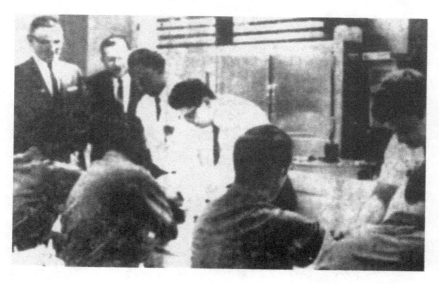

Superintendent Hendrick (at far left) observes technicians perform medical studies on prisoners. (February 1966) (© Urban Archives, Temple University, Philadelphia, PA)

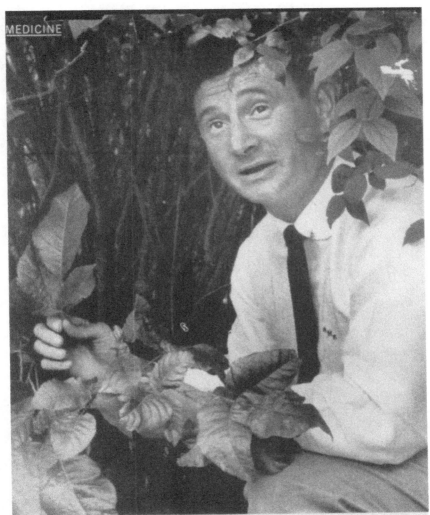

MEDICINE

NG POISON-FILLED LEAVES, DR. KLIGMAN COLLECTS TEST MATERIAL. ONCE HYPERSENSITIVE TO IVY, HE GETS ONLY MILD RASH SINCE USING

POISON IVY PICKER OF PENNYPACK PARK

Albert M. Kligman pictured in a 1955 *Life* magazine photoessay, glibly titled "Poison Ivy Picker of Pennypack Park." The caption reads, "Plucking poison-filled leaves, Dr. Kligman collects test material. Once hypersensitive to ivy, he gets only a mild rash since using vaccine." Kligman is one of the few dermatology professors to attract national media attention. This article and accompanying photos focus on his poison ivy experiments at Holmesburg.

(© Marvin Koner, originally appeared in *Life* Magazine, September 5, 1955)

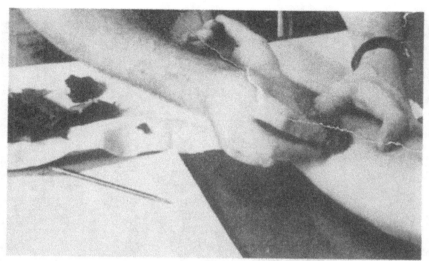

"APPLYING POISON to arm of a convict volunteer at Holmesburg Prison, an assistant rubs the crushed ivy leaves briskly to spread the toxic sap."

As the article states, these experiments gave "farmers and suburbanites reason to hope for the first practical ivy immunizer before the poisoning season of 1956." (© Marvin Koner, *Life* 1955)

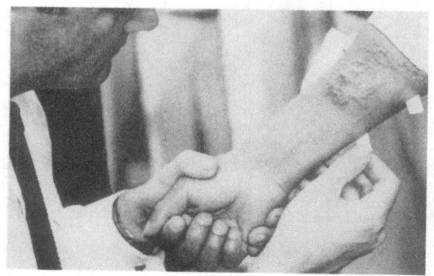

"ITCHY RASH appears on a convict who was not yet immunized. Before injections a small spot on each volunteer is poisoned to judge his sensibility."

As the caption indicates, each prisoner was first exposed to poison ivy before he could participate in the experiments. (© Marvin Koner, *Life* 1955)

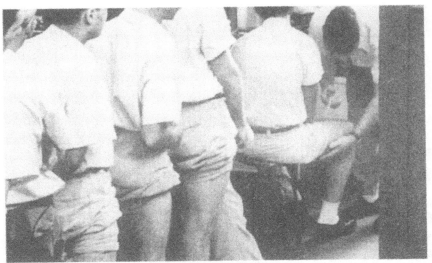

"GETTING IMMUNIZED, a group of convicts forms a line to get shots in thigh. Volunteers are plentiful since each man gets $2 or more for every shot."

According to *Life*, prisoners were "injected seven to 15 times" with a vaccine containing "a synthetic version of the poison in ivy's sap." No information is offered on whether the vaccine has been tested before or on what possible side-effects may be caused by so many injections. (© Marvin Koner, *Life* 1955)

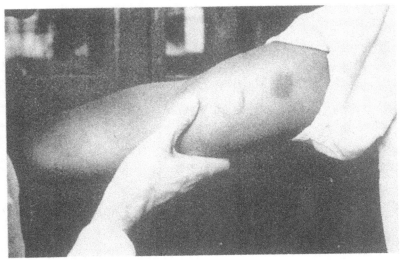

"VACCINE'S VALUE is seen when poison produces only discolored spots on the upper arm of a testee. Formerly this man was a highly sensitive victim."

Considering the prisoners as victims for participating in these tests is clearly unthinkable. (© Marvin Kolner, *Life* 1955)

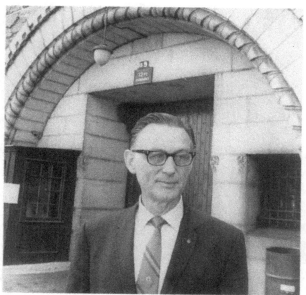

Edward Hendrick, Superintendent of the Philadelphia
Prison System. Throughout his lengthy career, Hendrick
allowed the medical experiments on prisioners. Pictured
at the Holmesburg Prison front gate in 1970. (© Urban
Archives, Temple University, Philadelphia, PA)

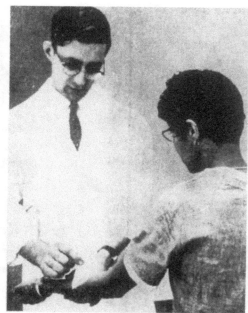

Dermatological patch tests were one of the
most common experiments at Holmesburg. A
medical technician examines the arm of an
inmate for irritation. (© Urban Archives, Temple
University, Philadelphia, PA)

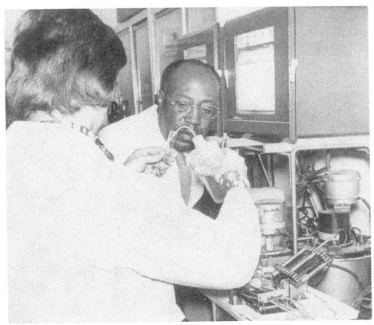

Solomon McBride, medical administrator of the Holmesburg human research program, observes a technician doing studies on fat content and cholesterol in humans. Shown in March of 1973, one year before the program would be shut down. (© Urban Archives, Temple University, Philadelphia, PA)

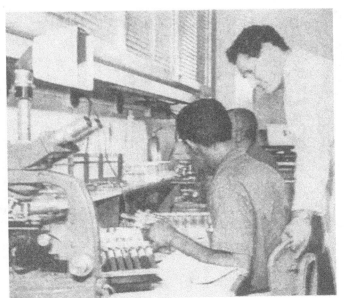

Prisoners performed varied roles in the research program. In February of 1966, two supervised inmates check blood slides in the hematology laboratory. (© Urban Archives, Temple University, Philadelphia, PA)

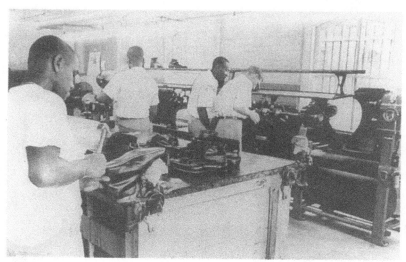

For the few lucky enough to earn a job, Holmesburg Prison's shoe shop offered prisoners long days and low wages. (September 1963) (© Urban Archives, Temple University, Philadelphia, PA)

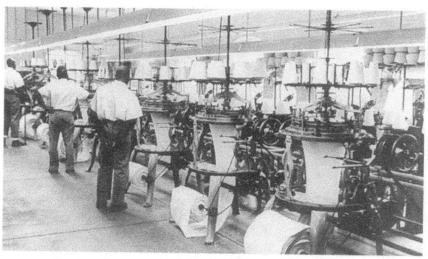

Holmesburg's knit-goods mill required few workers. Men choosing medical experiments earned considerably more than those few making shoes and clothing. (September 1963) (© Urban Archives, Temple University, Philadelphia, PA)

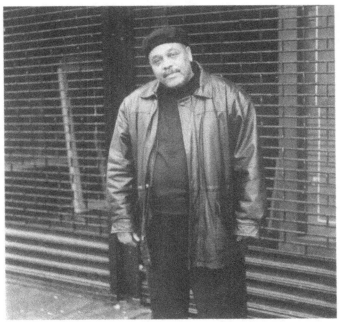

Leotis Jones participated in the experiments during the 1960s, but led the fight to end the testing program by testifying at U.S. senate hearings and later suing for legal damages. (Collection of the author, 1997)

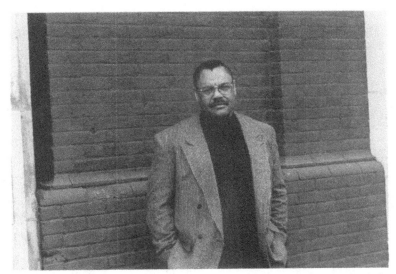

Thomas Sims said many inmate test subjects were skeptical of the strange ointments doctors placed on them. When they returned to their cell from H Block, it was not uncommon for prisoners to hang the adhesive bandages to their cell walls. (Collection of the author, 1997)

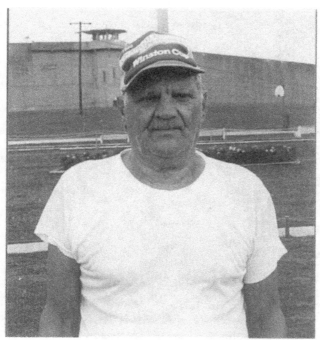

Withers Ponton, who recently died, endured dozens of experiments during his three years at Holmesburg. In need of money, each morning he went to H Block and asked, "Do you need me today?" (Collection of the author, 1995)

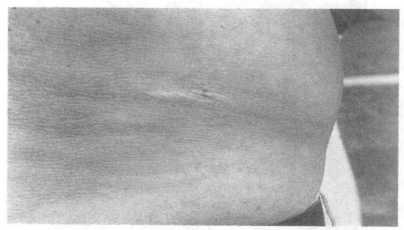

Inmate Ponton allowed the research program to use him as a human pin cushion. Two inch scars on each side of his abdomen are remnants of incisions doctors made for gauze implants that paid Ponton "$10 for each cut."(Collection of the author, 1995)

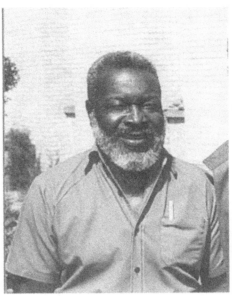

Matthew Epps worked as an intake interviewer for the research program and tried
to tell test volunteers "what experiments
to stay away from." (Collection of the author,
1995)

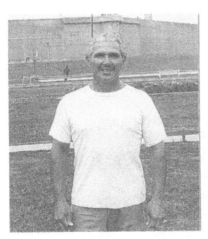

Al Zabala was initially afraid to participate in the experiments, but the
U.S. Army's chemical warfare studies offered "big money." His "good
trip" took him back to his youth.
(Collection of the author, 1995)

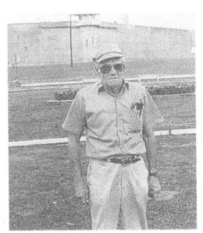

William McCafferty began his first
prison sentence in 1950. As the
inmate-nurse at Holmesburg, he
witnessed the early years of Dr.
Kligman's and the University of
Pennsylvania's human research program. McCafferty died in 1997; this
photo was taken in 1995. (Collection of
the author, 1995)

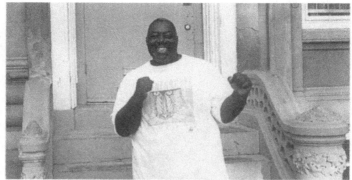

Roy "Tiger" Williams, a former ranked heavyweight boxer, lost his hair when he submitted to "a new dandruff shampoo experiment." (Collection of the author, 1994)

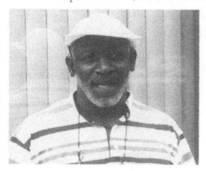

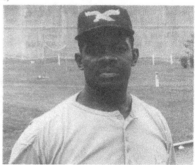

As a skilled jailhouse lawyer, Allan Lawson could earn money without subjecting himself to medical experiments. He was one of only two inmates to testify before a U.S. Senate Committee on prisoner experimentation. (Collection of the author, 1994)

A practicing Muslim, Simon Khaadim Ahad distrusted the doctors and their strange experiments. He encouraged others at Holmesburg not to participate in the "dangerous" practice. (Collection of the author, 1994)

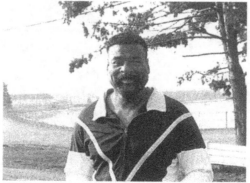

"Everyone did it for money," says former Holmesburg inmate Raymond Crawford of the experiments. Crawford rejected "the guinea pig situation. It just wasn't worth the chance." (Collection of the author, 1994)

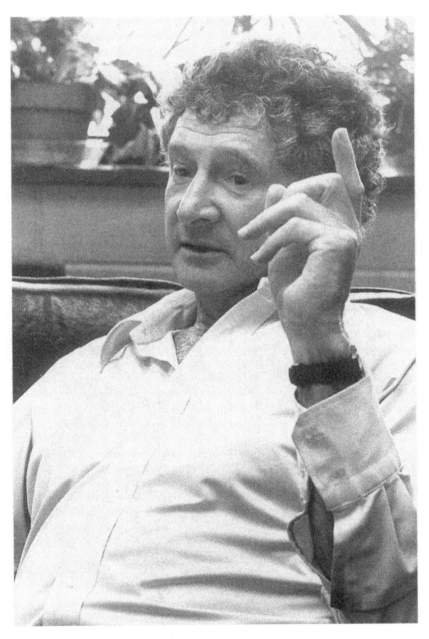

Dr. Kligman in his office in 1976, two years after the Holmesburg experiments were terminated. (© Urban Archives, Temple University, Philadelphia, PA)

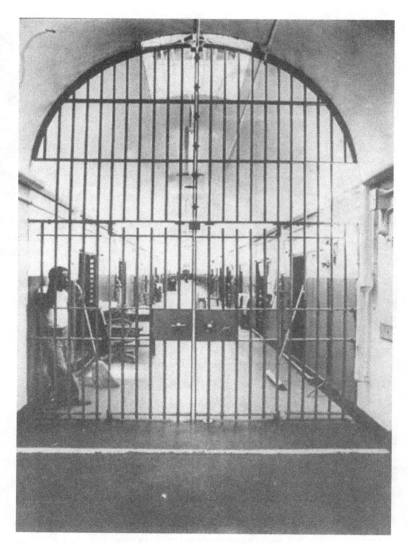

Several years after the Holmesburg experiments ended, H Block is pictured here in the late 1970s, once again serving as a housing block for prisoners. Holmesburg Prison was closed in December of 1995.
(© Urban Archives, Temple University, Philadelphia, PA)

"controlled environment," which was "quite desirable," prisoners were ideal subjects. For those fortunate enough to establish and maintain clinical testing programs in large institutions, Calesnick says, "It was like a gold mine."

The phone call from the AEC on October 19, 1964, was followed by a letter from the AEC confirming that a By-Product Material License was issued to the Holmesburg County Prison on January 2, 1964.[24] The license listed Dr. Calesnick as the authorized user. Calesnick wrote back immediately and informed the AEC that he had been asked to act as a "consultant to use or supervise the use of by-product materials" at Holmesburg. "However, since I have received no direct or indirect communications from that institution since this license was issued, I urgently request that my name be removed immediately as the authorized user" on the license.[25]

The uncertain role of Dr. Calesnick in the radioisotope program at Holmesburg is not unique. Arthur Wase, Ph.D., was also listed on Kligman's AEC application as the Isotope Safety Committee's "nucleonics advisor."[26] On October 29, 1964, Dr. Wase also sent a letter to the AEC, informing them that his "affiliation" with the Holmesburg isotope program had "ended in September, 1964."[27] He, too, requested that "if my name is included on the license or the application, it should be deleted since I am not a part of the program." Curiously, Dr. Kligman was still able to acquire the valuable license from the AEC even though the two key operatives who had the training and experience with radioactivity were no longer part of, if they had ever been, the proposed material license application.

IV

The Holmesburg protocols in the AEC file illuminate more of the story. In the AEC's Medical Advisory Committee response to Kligman's first 1963 protocol and application, the committee raised the problematic issue of using "prisoners for experimental work."[28] As one physician on the panel commented, "In view of the fact that a great deal has been written about prisoners for experimental work, and in view of the fact that this is going to be carried on at the Holmesburg County Prison, I have a strong suspicion that the Commission is wise in asking for a statement from the authorities of that prison as to their policy concerning this type of study on prisoners." Shortly thereafter, the AEC's Division of Licensing and Regulation wrote the Holmesburg Prison and requested "a statement from an official of your institution agreeing to have radioactive material on the premise and a statement concerning the use of radioactive materials on prisoners at the institution."[29]

In late October 1963, H. Earle Tucker, medical director of the Philadelphia prisons and "acting for Mr. Edward J. Hendrick, Superintendent," wrote back:

> We agree to have radioactive material on the premise at Holmesburg Prison and we are permitting the use of such material in testing programs involving prisoners at that institution because we have been assured by Dr. A. M. Kligman that the amounts used will be infinitesimal and the risks are essentially zero. In addition, the entire program will be supervised by a committee headed by Dr. Benjamin Calesnick, who will be directly responsible to Dr. A. M. Kligman.[30]

Several months later in January of 1964, the AEC granted Holmesburg Prison a license to store and use radioactive material. The license was to remain active for two years and expire on January 31, 1966. Several "conditions" for the license were enumerated, including the stipulation that "by-product material shall be used by, or under the supervision of, Benjamin Calesnick, M.D."[31]

Then, in October of 1964, Dr. Calesnick received the phone call that alerted him to the misuse of his name. He immediately notified the AEC, who amended Holmesburg's license in December 1964 to read: "By-product material shall be stored under the supervision of A. M. Kligman, M.D."[32] In a cover letter the AEC notified Kligman that with Dr. Calesnick's withdrawal as authorized user, "No person is authorized to use, or supervise the use of radiopharmaceuticals" under this license.[33] Furthermore, "If an amendment to the license is sought to add an authorized user, the technical qualifications of this person must be established."

On July 27, 1965, Dr. Kligman submitted a new application with a cover letter that said: "Changes in personnel and the direction of our studies under [the previous license] have been such that we are submitting a completely revised application for [an amendment to the] license suited to our current needs."[34] He reduced the number of isotopes to four, he left blank the section identifying the radiation protection officer, and he listed himself as the authorized user. The Isotope Safety Committee of the 1963 application became the Medical Isotope Committee whose members were Albert M. Kligman, M.D., certified dermatologist, and Herbert W. Copelan, M.D., internist.[35] The agency requested "information on Dr. A. M. Kligman's basic and clinical radioisotope training and experience," and on October 25, 1965, notified him that unless they received a response within 30 days, they would consider the application abandoned. On November 2, 1965 Dr. Kligman submitted his qualifications as authorized user. He reported that he had taken his technical training in 1963 in a six-month formal course under Dr. B. Calesnick at Hahnemann Hospital. He described his experience as two years of investigational use of radioisotopes at Hahnemann Hospital and Holmesburg Prison. The AEC accepted his qualifications, and requested his protocol for peer review by the Medical Advisory Committee. Dr. Calesnick firmly disputes Kligman's claim: "I never taught Kligman anything," he says. "Certainly not about radioactive material and never at Hahnemann. He never took any training program here of any length."[36] Calesnick is amazed that Kligman could make such claims and that the AEC could accept them so easily.

In March 1966, Kligman forwarded his protocol entitled "Studies of Human Epidermal Turnover Time Using S^{35} Cystine and H^3 Thymidine and of Cutaneous Permeability Using C^{14} Testosterone and Corticosteroid." This document specifies that "the subjects in these studies will be volunteer, male inmates...at Holmesburg of 21 to 50 years of age."[37] In addition, "Each subject signs a permission form showing his awareness of the nature of the experiment" that will entail the injection and application of radioactive materials. The protocol estimates that "for each of the materials under study...a maximum of 50 subjects will be required to obtain satisfactory data"—a potential total of 200 subjects. The human body's absorption and excretion rate for each of the materials is discussed with the assurance that "the applicant's training and experience in dermatology support the opinion that the dose from this technique will not have a significant likelihood of deleterious effect to the subject."

Panel members of the AEC's Medical Advisory Committee disagreed. Four of the seven reviewers disapproved the use of thymidine (H^3). One physician reviewing the protocol wrote, "This material, when injected, may reach the genetic DNA pool."[38] Another reviewer cautioned, "[I] don't think this experiment warrants possible hazard."[39] A third said that "information showing [that] the labeled compound remains in the tissue biopsy [and is not spread to others parts of the body] is essential before I would approve for human use."[40] And Dr. R. W. Rawson, who had raised the caution in 1963 about experimentation with prisoners, flatly disapproved "H3 as thymidine."[41] In May of 1966, the AEC granted Kligman an amendment to his materials license, limiting him to Carbon[14] and Sulfur.

Two years later on April 25, 1968, Kligman once again applied to amend and renew his by-product materials license. Once again he reported that his experience and training were obtained under the supervision of Benjamin Calesnick, M.D.[42] This time, Kligman added the isotope Sodium[22] (Na^{22}) in chloride. In additional skin-hardening tests he planned to inject the radioactive agents intradermally and then monitor the effect through the use of a gas flow chamber. In Kligman and Copelan's May 1967 annual report to the Army, the doctors stated that in an effort to gauge "cellular defense" patterns, "tritiated H^3-thymidine" was used along with numerous other staining agents, but the doctors concluded "that the specialized histochemical stains have not yielded information proportionate to the effort" and abandoned the test.[43] (Of course, Kligman had also been denied any further use of H^3.) Little else was mentioned regarding the use of radioactive materials in these 1966–67 experiments, but the doctors informed the military of plans for future studies—evidently involving the use of Sodium[22].

When Paul Goldberg, the operations branch project manager of the AEC's Division of Industrial and Medical Nuclear Safety, is asked about Calesnick's and Wase's early withdrawal from the Holmesburg application, he says that "no other example comes to mind...of physicians declaring uninvolvement."[44] As to the agency's mandate that properly trained individuals supervise radioactive material, Goldberg does not waiver. "We would [have insisted] on a licensed medical person trained or experienced in radioactive materials. There had to be a radioactive safety officer as an authorized user of the by-product material."

V

One of the few doctors willing to discuss his Holmesburg years and the use of radioactive materials is Dr. Issac Willis. The former chairman of Morehouse College's department of dermatology claims that he and his colleagues were very careful, but fell far short of current standards.[45] Dr. Willis, who was a resident at the University of Pennsylvania in the mid- and late 1960s, attempts to mitigate the potential risks of using radioactive materials by saying that those substances were in "very little" use at Holmesburg and usually "at the very end" of an experiment. Willis refers to thymidine, the H^3 isotope approved in Kligman's first application in 1963 and disapproved in the 1965 amendment. Willis says that when thymidine was "injected," it was usually "excised within minutes" and was never "left for any length of time" in the subject's body. "[We would] take it out before it was absorbed. I never participated in any experiments where thymidine was left in the body for any length of time." In addition, he explains, "Zylocaine and ephedrine were used to control the thymidine [and] limit its spread." Stressing his own professional rectitude during his years of research at Holmesburg, Willis admits, "We can't take what happened there casually...if thymidine had gotten into an inmate's bloodstream, it would have been very bad."

As for the other prison experiments, Dr. Willis claims he had very little knowledge of them. "The military experiments were done in such secrecy that I didn't know they were taking place....I didn't have the foggiest idea that people were being exposed to warfare chemicals." Nevertheless, Willis knew enough to be able to make comparisons; he reports that the tests he administered paid the inmates "virtually nothing compared to the Army experiments," but Willis's group was never short of volunteers. "We were very popular. Some other experiments had a definite reputation, but the studies I worked on were perceived as not very dangerous."

Although he is obviously uncomfortable looking back on his

Six

"Danger! This Material Is *Extremely* Toxic."

I

Ordinarily, he would thumb through the magazine while he killed time and pick up bits of information. *Corrections* magazine had become a staple of casual reading for the convicts at Graterford State Penitentiary in Montgomery County, just west of Philadelphia. On this day, however, Al Zabala, in and out of jail for the last fifteen years, would pay close attention to an article in the April 1981 issue. "As soon as I seen it, I knew they were talking about me," said Zabala. "I knew everything they were saying in the article."[1]

Almost everything. For the first time, Zabala learned the name of a dangerous chemical—dioxin—to which he may have been exposed. The trade magazine contained an eye-catching story about unusual medical experiments that had been performed at a county prison in Philadelphia during the mid-1960s. Zabala read with interest and felt his heart begin to race; the article hit close to home.

Zabala hated and avoided writing letters, but the article advised contacting the Environmental Protection Agency (EPA), so he wrote that he had been at Holmesburg Prison in 1964 and 1965, and thought that he had been part of the dioxin experiments. He added that "the reason why no one can come up with any records is they all were destroyed by the prison, Dow Chemical, and the University of Pennsylvania." He argued that the doctors knew "they would have legal problems at a later date" and decided to deep-six the evidence.[2]

Zabala's letter did not surprise the EPA, which had received a flood of correspondence from concerned inmates and former prisoners ever since the story had broken earlier in the year. Under the banner headline of the January 11, 1981, Sunday edition of the *Philadelphia Inquirer*, "Human Guinea Pigs: Dioxin Tested at Holmesburg," a front-page article described how a corporation (Dow Chemical) and a university (University of Pennsylvania) joined together to test a dangerous chemical substance on the backs of Holmesburg Prison inmates.[3] Nearly six dozen inmates had been purposely exposed to something formally known as 2, 3, 7, 8–tetrachloro-p-dibenzodioxin, or TCDD, a by-product of the manufacture of the herbicide 2, 4, 5-T. The substance had been "linked by scientists to cancer, birth defects and fetal cancer," and a Harvard professor was quoted as saying that dioxin may be "the most powerful carcinogen known" to man.[4]

The lengthy article made several interesting points: Dr. Kligman, the orchestrator of the experiments, was paid $10,000 for his services; the experiment may have been the only instance in which the level of exposure of humans to dioxin was known; the test subjects could be suffering long-term health effects that, if discovered in time, might be possible to arrest; and the current health of the subjects could provide valuable evidence in the bitter debate over whether herbicides containing dioxin are safe.

The government's growing concern about the health effects of widespread use of herbicides that contained dioxin had led to greater restrictions but not total prohibitions. Rice fields and range land were still the sites of periodic disseminations of 2, 4, 5-T and silvex to destroy unwanted vegetation, and silvex was still being used on some fruit orchards. The EPA proposed to ban all uses of 2, 4, 5-T and silvex. Dow Chemical adamantly opposed a ban. It was this impasse that fostered the Holmesburg revelations. Manufacturing at least half of the nation's supply of 2, 4, 5-T, Dow was not going to give up its valuable product without a fight. Their spokesman at hearings in Washington, D.C., in late 1980, was Verald Keith Rowe, a career official at Dow.

II

On November 13, 1980, Mr. Rowe, a consultant to the vice president for health and environmental sciences at the Dow Chemical Company testified before the EPA. A 43-year veteran of the giant chemical company, Rowe had risen through the ranks, and as the assistant director of the Biochemical Research Laboratory in the mid-1960s, his career had intersected with the history of human experimentation at Holmesburg Prison. By 1973, Rowe had become the director of toxicological affairs and health and environmental research. He had retired from the company six years later, but was still retained as a consultant.

Rowe told the panel that an unexpected outbreak of chloracne ("a skin disease characterized by an eruption of blackheads in a highly distinctive pattern") among the workers at Dow's Midland, Michigan, 2, 4, 5-T plant in 1964 had caused considerable concern. The plant was closed immediately, various governmental agencies were notified, and a series of tests were begun to determine the cause. The company believed that 49 workers had developed chloracne as a result of a change in the reaction process at the 2, 4, 5-T plant. The contaminant appeared to be the waste generated by the manufacturing process, and further testing isolated 2, 3, 7, 8-TCDD as the chemical impurity and probable cause of the chloracne. Animal tests were begun using a rabbit-ear bioassay, a comparison of the biological activity produced by 2, 3, 7, 8-TCDD with the effects of a standard substance. The results, according to Rowe, showed that "0.2 micrograms was without effect on the rabbit ear; 0.5 micrograms usually caused a positive response; and 4–8 micrograms usually caused a severe response."[5]

Understandably, company toxicologists wanted to compare the effects produced by TCDD in rabbit ears to the effects produced in humans. Rowe said that "to help answer this question, [he] contacted Dr. Albert Kligman, a professor of dermatology at the University of Pennsylvania, who was known to have tested the safety of various chemicals and drugs in volunteers from a prison in Lewisburg, Pennsylvania."[6] Although he had confused Holmesburg with the federal penitentiary in northcentral Pennsylvania, Rowe got the right man. "Dr. Kligman agreed to test the chloracnegenic potential of TCDD in humans under his existing program."

According to an internal Dow memorandum from Rowe to 10 high-ranking company officials, Dr. Kligman visited the company's Michigan headquarters on December 11, 1964, and listened to a presentation of Dow's chloracne problem. Kligman responded within two weeks with a "proposed program for a basic study on acne."[7]

Rowe encouraged his research colleagues to accept the offer by stating: "We need to know the quantitative as well as the qualitative relationships between the sensitivity of the rabbit and man." He also believed that the company needed "to know something about the basic changes that occur in the skin in response to given acnegens...the effects of these materials upon the microflora of the skin and what, if any, treatments it begins to develop." Rowe pointed out that "Dr. Kligman is very desirous of searching for the answer to these questions," and "it would be our intention to correlate his work on humans with rabbit work done here with exactly the same compositions."[8]

In early March of 1965, Rowe requested "authorization for $10,000 for research on chemical acnegens using human subjects."[9] He stated that he would "like to have the approval" of the directors of research and production so that Kligman's "proposed study" could commence. As an incentive, he passed along a copy of a Kligman communication that "relieved the Company of any liability which may be incurred by [the] experimental work."

It is unclear whether Dow requested the release or Kligman offered it to sweeten the financial contract, but on March 2, 1965, Kligman had sent Rowe a letter stating that "the Dow Chemical Company is released from liability in case of adverse effects developing in human volunteers in the course of certain studies in which the Dow Chemical Company is interested."[10] Kligman confidently wrote, "I assume full responsibility for any liabilities which may arise in connection with human testing," because his operation had "never encountered a problem in this respect." Moreover, Kligman added, all his "contracts with industry" provided similar terms.

Eight days later, Kligman responded to a Dow request for a copy of his "Permission to Perform Tests." This waiver, intended for prisoners to sign as consent for testing, contained a simple, single sentence stated: "I, the undersigned, also hereby give my permission to the hospital, laboratories or others to perform medical and other tests on me: the hospital, laboratories, etc. or the prison are not to be held responsible in any way for any complications or untoward results that may arise."[11]

Three months later, on July 9, 1964, Rowe sent Kligman an experimental protocol and a sample of 2, 3, 7, 8-tetrachloro-p-dibenzodioxin (TCDD) described as "a potent acnegen" and "highly toxic."[12] Kligman was warned that oral doses of the chemical had proved deadly to rabbits and at the very least had produced "severe liver and kidney injury." Rowe said "it [did] not seem probable" that his proposed protocol would present a "serious systemic hazard" to Kligman's volunteers since on a per kilogram basis it was less than what produced "any significant effect...in the rabbit." "Nevertheless," emphasized Rowe, "the seriousness of the type of consequences that might develop from testing with this...compound require that we approach the matter in a highly conservative manner." In accordance with his concern, Rowe recommended that they use just two inmate-volunteers to begin the experiment, and test over the course of several months. This, he argued, would be the "safe way to proceed," but he let Kligman know that "the number of persons in your experiment, is your decision." The protocol recommended observation periods, test substance solubility, and the progressively rising doses that the subject should receive, ranging from 0.2 to 8.0 in strength. Rowe also stated in his letter that all related solutions should be labeled with the warning: "Danger! This material is *extremely* toxic."

III

Thus began the first scientifically monitored tests of TCDD in humans. The experiment started in late 1965 and was completed in early 1966. In May 1966, Dr. Kligman sent Dow a final report, describing "the astonishingly negative results."[13] Rowe was informed "that the human is far more resistant to acnegenic substances than the rabbit ear" and it was now apparent that "prolonged contact is necessary to produce chemical acne in humans." Kligman said he now realized "that relatively high concentrations and chronic exposure" would be necessary, and asked Dow for "another year" so that the original program could be carried out. He explained that his "general study" of the causes of human acne vulgaris had intensified, and claimed "one of these days we are going to shine a light into this cave." Once again he requested that Dow stay the course and told Rowe, "I am greatly in need of your support."

Kligman included a brief synopsis of the initial six-month study that had subjected ten inmates to progressive doses on their foreheads and backs. Obviously dismayed, he described the experiment as "thoroughly negative" since "none of the subjects developed acne." Foreshadowing what was to come, Kligman said, "I am hopeful that you will extend our grant for another year so that we can carry out our original program."[14]

The control substance used in the bioassay with humans was Dow Compound 6X, Hexachloral Diphenol Oxide, a "long-known potent chloracnegen." Though not dioxin, it could produce similar results.[15] Dow 6X was mixed in an assortment of vehicles including hexane, alcohol chloroform, ethylene glycol, and Carbowax. Concentrations ran from 1 percent to 10 percent and were applied either once or twice daily to the mid-back, forehead, forearm, and over the mastoid process behind the ear. Kligman informed the Michigan company that the results varied from "moderate irritation" to insignificant acne.[16] Rowe's testimony before the EPA provides a good summary of the similar procedure Kligman followed with the dioxin.

> Dr. Kligman reported that the subjects were divided into 6 separate groups of 10 each. The first group was studied in two phases: initially, a single dose of 0.2 microgram was administered; after a two week interval, the same total dose (0.2 microgram) was administered to the same skin site in two daily doses of 0.1 microgram. In half the subjects, the dose was administered to the forehead, in the other half the dose was administered to the mid-back region. The application site was covered for 24 hours by a 2-inch gauze square.
>
> One week after the single dose, and 3–4 days after the final daily dose, chemical tests were performed on each subject. These tests included CBC (hematology test), BUN and creatinine clearance (kidney function tests), and SGOT and alkaline phosphates (liver function tests). At the end of each phase, the subjects were examined by an internist for signs of systemic illness. The skin was examined weekly for six weeks after the last dose.
>
> Following the medical examination of the subjects in Group 1, the same procedure was repeated for Group 2, except [an] initial dose of 0.5 microgram [was] administered in daily applications of 0.1 microgram. Taking the initial and daily doses together, the total dose in Group 2 was 1.0 microgram. The same procedure was used for all the remaining Groups.[17]

Kligman ended his brief report by stating that "there was not the slightest bit of acne, either on the forehead or the back" and "no subject developed symptoms that could be related to the treatment." In short, Kligman found that at the recommended dosage level, "the test agent gave no evidence of being acnegenic and was not harmful to the subjects."[18]

Upon learning the results of Kligman's experiments, especially the lack of information about what dosage level formed the threshold that would produce chloracne in humans, Rowe indicated to Dr. Kligman that Dow would fund a continuation of his studies.

A year and a half later, in January 1968, Verald Rowe received a letter from the University of Pennsylvania dermatologist reporting new results. In his two-page letter, Kligman reported that the inability to establish a threshold for TCDD in the earlier test "encouraged me to proceed more vigorously."[19] He therefore had assembled another "panel of 10 subjects and applied 0.05 ML of a 1% solution in alcohol chloroform to a one inch square on the back." Applied every other day for a month, the new protocol achieved a positive result: "8 of 10 subjects showed acne form lesions...and 3 had lesions that progressed to inflammatory pustules and papules." The lesions lasted from 4 to 7 months, but their duration was obviously exacerbated by Kligman's decision that "no effort [should be] made to speed healing by active treatment."

Each week for six weeks the test subjects went through a battery of medical tests that reportedly resulted in "no instance of laboratory or clinical toxicity," other than the chloracne. "The subjects," Kligman wrote to Rowe, "remained well throughout the study."

The total dosage of dioxin given to the ten prisoners was 7,500 micrograms, an amount that astonished Rowe. "I remember writing the protocol," said Rowe in a recent interview.[20] "I started the protocol with low-dosage levels and increased it by small increments to indicate the slightest change in any physical reaction. The protocol I gave him was conservative...and very specific, but I had no control if he decided to change it." Rowe says the Dow scientists were "quite startled" when they saw that Kligman had dramatically altered the protocol by increasing the dosage 468 times.

"His protocol was quite amazing," says Rowe, "and it caused us to sever the relationship. If we couldn't get a straight deal, that caused us great trouble. He didn't give us any notice. That was the end of the relationship with Dr. Kligman."[21] Most disappointing for Dow, the three-year study never achieved the original goal. Although Dr. Kligman had informed his corporate client that "it is much more difficult to induce acne in the human than in the rabbit ear," he had not found the critical threshold dose.[22] Rowe said at the conclusion of his 1980 Washington testimony that Dr. Kligman's last experiment did "not permit the definition of a threshold exposure for the induction of chloracne by TCDD in man, as was my purpose in initiating the study."[23] The key dose fell somewhere between 16 micrograms and 7,500 micrograms, a considerable scientific gap.

At the conclusion of his EPA testimony, Rowe was asked a series of uncomfortable questions about Dow's lack of oversight on the dioxin experiments at Holmesburg. He said Kligman's second, more aggressive protocol was a "total surprise" and a radical departure from Rowe's own, more conservative approach. Dow, according to Rowe, had "had reasonable confidence that [Kligman] would proceed in a manner consistent with our original protocol." They had not seen a need for further instructions to Kligman before the start of the second protocol. When pressed about why Dow didn't keep closer tabs on Kligman's "laboratory work," Rowe said that the company had assumed that, as was their standard practice, they had hired "competent people" for the dioxin tests. He pointed out that Dr. Kligman was a professor of dermatology, "an M.D., he did lots and lots of skin work in those days."[24] In short, Rowe believed it unnecessary to look over the shoulder of an eminent physician and researcher in order to monitor his procedure. Dow had never imagined that Kligman would exercise such unorthodox zeal contrary to the company's specific protocol.

Thirty years after the unusual human experiments, Rowe still clearly recalls the answers to the critical questions surrounding the Holmesburg dioxin experiments. Why, for example, did an international industrial titan with its own sophisticated laboratory contract out lab work on its own product? Rowe simply states that Dow research personnel "were quite certain" that dioxin was the cause of the chloracne in their workers, but "wanted [their] findings confirmed." They knew that the manufacture of the herbicide 2, 4, 5-T led to dioxin as a by-product. Dow's "protocol was for documentation" purposes. Though lab work was rarely contracted out, Rowe says: "Dr. Albert Kligman was a well-known dermatologist" who did human testing "so we went to him." Why, when for years Upjohn and Parke-Davis had been using hundreds of prisoners for experimentation purposes at the Michigan State Penitentiary in Jackson, did a Michigan-based company with in-state academic talent turn to a Pennsylvania university and prison to perform such experiments? Rowe responds simply: "I didn't know of the Michigan prison tests."

To the questions of why African-American prisoners were represented in disproportionate numbers in the dioxin experiments (47 to 9 in the first protocol), and why Dow accepted such a minimal document as evidence of informed consent, Rowe has no answers. But he seems undisturbed by either the unbalanced racial composition of the test population or the prisoners' degree of informed consent. Rowe says, "I don't have too much of a problem with Kligman's operation in that regard." He makes clear that such items were the preserve of Dr. Kligman. "The protocol was my business. I knew what I wrote and what I wanted."[25]

IV

Rowe's unexpected testimony at the EPA hearings was widely covered by the media and created considerable public interest and repercussions. A cross-section of normally divergent constituencies became fascinated with the callous prison experiment. At the head of the line were the inmates themselves, men who had been subjected to a host of experiments, particularly the frequent patch tests that were identical to the dioxin studies in the procedure.

On learning that EPA investigators were searching for participants in the Holmesburg dioxin studies, numerous former and current prisoners responded (particularly those who were daily newspaper readers). The letters were quite similar in expressing their concern, describing their years at Holmesburg, and requesting more information. The following letters were obtained through the Freedom of Information Act. One dated January 12, 1981, a day after the revealing article appeared in the *Philadelphia Inquirer,* begins:

I believe I was one of those inmates at Holmesburg Prison at the time those tests were being done on the inmates....I have had tests done on my back, forearm, and I believe a hair test as well. In the later part of the sixties, I had a reaction to something but I never did learn why I had foam at the mouth like I had rabies or something. Also two marks on my left forearm are still quite visible. [26]

Another began:

I was a prisoner in Holmesburg in 1967 and injected with dioxin as part of a medical testing program there. We were supposed to get money or time off for participating in these tests. I was given injections every 10 days, following a pattern of different colors that were patches on my arm and shoulders and matched with the colors on the card....Six or seven other prisoners were injected with me at one time. We were injected once a week for five or six weeks. [27]

The former inmate concluded his testimony by describing his declining health which included: progressively worsening eyesight and the need for "new glasses about every year for the past 11 to 12 years," "a white smelly substance" emanating from the pores on his nose, behind his ears, and his forehead, and a chronic nervous condition.

Newspapers around the country published articles about the Dow-Holmesburg experiments and generated inquiries from former prisoners outside the Philadelphia area. One writer in a Michigan prison wrote:

The Agent Orange article...was quite shocking. [The letter enclosed the article from the *Detroit Free Press* entitled "Agent Orange Component Tested on Convicts."[28]] I did two skin tests at Holmesburg Prison in 1968....The back test I was on for two weeks where a clear white fluid was rubbed on in different spots, usually lower back. I have no idea of the dosages applied or what the fluid was. The medical personnel told the guys on the test this was a skin softener test. Some guys had numerous biopsies taken all over their back, they were paid $25 for each biopsy taken. I refused the biopsy. The paper work we signed for permission to test was kept by the medical personnel. We were not given copies of agreements nor any receipts on these tests. [29]

On occasion, nonparticipants wrote expressing concern about their friends: "The purpose of this letter is to inform you of the name and location of one of those guinea pigs. My dearest friend and I were inmates at Holmesburg during that time, and he participated in the testing programs, over my most strenuous objections."[30]

The inmates' concerns were given added weight and impetus by the growing controversy surrounding the use of Agent Orange in Southeast Asia. Thousands of Vietnam veterans charged the government and large chemical companies with assorted crimes arising out of the production and use of Agent Orange. (The key ingredient of Agent Orange and the herbicide 2, 4, 5-T was dioxin.) The veterans firmly believed that the chemical was the source of their mysterious health problems that ranged from festering sores and malignant tumors to birth defects and stillbirths. The former GIs argued that the Air Force had sprayed more than 19 million gallons of Agent Orange to defoliate 5 million acres of Vietnamese countryside, and that their own exposure had led directly to their medical problems.

Various governmental agencies denied the accusations, but the Holmesburg revelations offered an opportunity to resolve the debate. For the first time, apparently, human beings had received measured and scientifically monitored doses of dioxin. It was hoped that military doctors might now be in the position to determine the biological effects of Agent Orange, and civilian doctors the effects of exposure to herbicides. Dow remained adamant, however, that there was no concrete evidence linking health defects to dioxin. Even though 2, 4, 5,-T represented only $14 million of the company's annual sales, which in 1979 exceeded $9 billion, Dow said a "scientific principle" was at stake. They argued that for more than 30 years the product had been tested and retested, more so "than most drugs found in your medicine cabinet. The preponderance of data demonstrates that 2, 4, 5-T does not pose an unreasonable risk."[31] While the military remained firm that Agent Orance had caused no ill-effects to the soldiers in Vietnam, the EPA remained equally firm in its belief that herbicides spread on pastures, farmlands, and forests could promote stillbirths, birth defects, and cancer. The EPA believed that there were no safe levels of dioxin exposure.

V

Into this cauldron of competing interests came the potential to collect unprecedented data from the Holmesburg inmates who had participated in the dioxin experiments. But could the EPA find them? Dr. Kligman and the prison system claimed the relevant paperwork had been discarded and destroyed years earlier. Out of the hundreds who over a 20-year span had taken part in various experiments, the administrators said they no longer knew who had participated in the dioxin tests.

Follow-up newspaper articles informed the public that the EPA planned to send "medical investigators to Philadelphia to interview worried residents who feared they may have been exposed to a highly toxic component of Agent Orange" years earlier.[32] But investigators cautioned that they had "little prospect of establishing which inmates were the subject of the dioxin tests" because of "lost or destroyed" records.

One outspoken critic who was quoted in the same article was Dr. Sigmund Weitzman, at the time a cancer specialist at Massachusetts General Hospital in Boston. "It is important," he argued, "for government to follow these people to know the true consequences" of researchers' actions.[33] Cancer, he pointed out, might not become apparent for another five to ten years. In a 1994 interview with the author, Weitzman goes further. He is furious that records of the people exposed to toxic substances were not kept. He calls such lax research practices "unconscionable" and "disgraceful."[34]

Dr. Weitzman, who was introduced in chapter 1, is more than a detached scientific observer. He had been a 22-year-old medical student and technician at Holmesburg in the summer of 1967, when the dioxin tests were underway. He recalls getting "so mad" when he read the 1981 newspaper article and says it was "just awful and incredible...exposing [the inmates] and not telling them what they were testing. It's horrible. I was told we were testing commercial products prior to marketing,....I didn't know what [they] were [but] it wasn't Chanel they were testing on the prisoners. All the people who were doing the testing were splashed and exposed on a daily basis without being aware [of the precise chemical], and they would be at high risk." He says, "Naturally, I'm concerned about my own health, too....I'm not sure whether I was exposed to dioxin." [35]

Dr. Weitzman reserves his most critical comments for the testing program's chief. "Kligman only cared about his own work. It was purely for money, there was nothing scientific about it. You would keep your data if it was serious science. In science, you keep your [data]." Weitzman wonders out loud "how a man so eminent, with a universal reputation, could be involved in such stuff?"

Although Dr. Kligman declined all newspaper interviews at the time, one article mentioned his response to a television interview, in which he claimed the experiments were quite innocuous and the amount of applied dioxin was "so small that you couldn't see it on the end of your fingernail."[36] Kligman added that the "imputations" of "padded cells," "CIA" involvement, and other assorted crimes were "outrageous." In unintended irony, Kligman said angrily, "Christ, it sounds like Nazi Germany."

Some of the inmates agreed. Another front-page story told of Robert Crew and Earl Harris, "2 Men Scarred for Life" after being subjected to Holmesburg "hot patch tests."[37] The article discussed profiteering by lab workers and recurring inmate body rashes that no one had been able to cure. "To look back at it now, it was an atrocity. We never knew what they were using on us," said Crew. "We just asked how much did it pay. That was the first thing we asked. Now you see what the Germans were doing experimenting on humans. It's the same thing they were doing to us, with just a little more diplomacy."

VI

For the Environmental Protection Agency, the January 1981 newspaper headlines proved more burdensome than the original Dow testimony the previous November. Reporters as well as prisoners were now asking what the EPA planned to do about the Holmesburg human guinea pigs. Minority newspapers, in particular, played up the racial implications of the human research program. The *Philadelphia Tribune* devoted several front-page news articles to the "guinea pigs" story, including "painful" personal tales by the test subjects themselves.[38] One inmate called it "a clear case of genocide," since the "inhuman experiments" were practiced on a prison population that was "over-whelmingly black and non-white." No longer, the inmate warned, should people doubt or dismiss the "covert, as well as overt genocidal game being run on Black folks."[39] Another *Tribune* story told the sad tale of James "Jimbo" Willis, a former "prison guinea pig" who never fully recovered from his Holmesburg experience and was eventually killed by police in a violent street confrontation.[40]

A full-scale investigation seemed necessary, but some at the EPA feared the potential scope and expense. In a January 29, 1981, memorandum, the director of the health effects branch told the deputy assistant administrator for pesticide programs that they were already dispatching health investigators to interview those "persons who have been identified as subjects of the TCDD studies," but stressed his belief that this effort is "not likely to result in data of immediate use to the Agency."[41] The director expressed deep "reservations about any substantive OPP (Office of Pesticide Programs) involvement" in the Holmesburg dioxin matter, and cautioned against "possible pitfalls [that] may arise from involvement in this issue."

He then listed several reasons why the EPA should undertake a measured, "low-key" response to the Holmesburg dioxin story, rather than the more thorough and in-depth investigation that many people expected. First was the belief that it would be "virtually impossible to conduct a dose-response analysis" of specific individuals because of the unavailability of the test records and the inability to establish "a matched control group" of former prisoners. Second, a "detailed physical examination" of each individual "would be quite resource intensive" and would most likely "cost in excess of $100,000." Third, the individuals examined would "understandably want...explanation[s] or interpretation[s] derived from their respective physicals," a further drain on the agency, and fourth, "any hint of an adverse effect" could lead to lawsuits and "further tax EPA resources in responding to the medics, Congress, etc."[42]

Other internal communications among various EPA departments during the winter and spring of 1981 reveal repeated recommendations to control and "clean up" this "extremely volatile issue" as soon as possible.[43] In early May, the EPA decided to narrow the scope of their investigation by abandoning a proposed "follow-up survey" of dioxin subjects and Holmesburg prisoners. By streamlining the process, one senior science advisor hoped to "clean this up within the next two or three weeks."[44] Less than a week later, EPA documents disclose the decision to take no further action on a lengthy questionnaire identifying those "individuals who participated in the Kligman/Dow dioxin testing."[45] The EPA gave the following reasons: U.S. Army experiments had been held at the same time as the Dow experiments and had also "resulted in the skin lesions"; Kligman had used "some prisoners in more than one test," making it virtually impossible to associate a particular health problem with a single chemical; the written records were gone; and the inmates' testimony was inadequate because they were "never aware of the chemical they were tested with."

Instead of pursuing the Holmesburg inmate-volunteers, the EPA decided to require that the former Holmesburg prisoners pursue the EPA. Under the guise of searching for former dioxin test subjects, the agency established three criteria, two of them hidden, for follow-up interviews. First, any inmate who believed himself to have been part of the dioxin experiments would be required to write the EPA. This was the only criteria that was publicized. An August 1981 EPA memo that began, "I hope everybody involved in this remembers that the purpose is to calm things down—not stir them up," explains what happened after the inmate wrote the EPA.[46] John W. Melone, the acting director of the Hazard Evaluation Division, told his colleagues that the "intent" of the interview process was to "test our hypothesis that a complete study would not be useful" because it appeared hopeless that the true dioxin subjects would be discovered. He said that of the 40 former inmates who had contacted the EPA and claimed dioxin exposure, only the "18 individuals residing in Philadelphia were sent letters which stated they were selected for the initial interviews." The Agency excluded 23 former Holmesburg inmates who were then incarcerated in ten prisons in eight different states.[47]

The agency did not intend to interview any former test subjects still in prison. Those unlucky men were sent one-page letters informing them that because of documentation difficulties, "we have decided to alter our previous approach" and only "a portion" of the subject pool would be interviewed. The letter informed the inmate that "you are not one of the individuals selected for the initial interview" and then thanked him for his "interest in this matter."[48]

Those former test subjects who were out of prison and residing in Philadelphia received letters that included the key passage, "You are one of the individuals selected." The letter then asked them to contact the EPA office by phone or mail,[49] at which time the former inmates were notified of their personal interviews to be held in Philadelphia on October 28–29, 1981. Of the 10 who formally made an appointment for an interview, 6 former inmates appeared. Three others were later interviewed by telephone. The environmental agency's minimalist approach to its investigtion of the dioxin experiments effectively limited the test subject pool to those who read the newspaper (eliminating the high percentage of Holmesburg inmates who were functional illiterates), were able to write the EPA, were out of prison, and living in Philadelphia.

VII

Frank L. Davido, the EPA's pesticide incident response officer, conducted the interviews that included "questionnaires and free flowing conversation."[50] He submitted an eight-page final report about the Holmesburg investigation. Coming almost one year after newspaper headlines had startled the general public and former test subjects about the true nature of the Holmesburg experiments, Davido informed his superiors "that none of the nine men interviewed could with certainty be said to have been involved in any dioxin testing." He claimed it was "not possible to accurately identify" the true dioxin subjects because of the host of reasons already known to the agency. Davido said the "only reliable method" of identification would have been through written record and "this approach was impossible." He pointed out that the investigation would not have been "any more successful" if 40 to 50 men had been interviewed, and he concluded his report by advising his office to "take no further investigative action on the dioxin experiments conducted at Holmesburg Prison."

In a recent interview Frank Davido, a 26-year EPA veteran, said the Dow-Kligman affair stands out in his mind because of the twin issues of prison inmates and human experimentation. He states, "I've been involved with different police forces and law enforcement agencies in tracking down different people or substances, but none where I had to track down prisoners who were exposed to toxic chemicals."[51] When asked why only 9 out of 75 prisoners were interviewed, Davido says that "it was proposed to visit the various prison systems, but later there was a decision to just visit those who were free and living outside of prison. I don't recall why we decided not to visit and interview incarcerated individuals." He defended the EPA decisions by arguing, "We were just trying to acquire information. We were after the science of the problem."

Despite believing that some of those inmates he interviewed were exposed to dioxin, he says the hard evidence that was necessary to substantiate their claims was not there. "I concluded that I couldn't prove that dioxin caused" their physical health problems, says Davido.

To the former Holmesburg human guinea pigs who had reached out to the EPA for help, the EPA's response was disheartening. Those who were still incarcerated remained unaware that their imprisonment excluded them from personal interviews and a greater understanding of their conditions. Many believed that their having signed waivers precluded access to any government recourse. Some, like Al Zabala, continued to write the EPA, only to receive ever briefer replies[52] and, in the end, a copy of Davido's final report.[53] Most let the matter drop, a not-unusual practice for prisoners fatalistic about their health and accustomed to harsh treatment from the government.

An EPA consultant recognized potential public relations problems in the final report, even though he agreed that "Frank Davido's analysis of the problem is sound, and his conclusion justified."[54] Dr. Donald P. Morgan of the University of Iowa's department of preventive medicine and environmental health advised the agency that "In a case such as this, you may want to be careful about impugning the credibility of these participants, especially when you can't prove your own conclusion." Dr. Morgan need not have worried. There was no uproar about the agency's findings; the plight of prisoners was not a high priority during the early years of the Reagan admin-istration. The EPA, as it had hoped, was able to extricate itself from a human tragedy of unknowable proportions. Fewer than four dozen former prisoners contacted the EPA—a pitifully small number out of the large pool of subjects that had participated in patch tests at Holmesburg.

The Holmesburg dioxin debacle receded from the public's con-sciousness except for periodic news articles published, for the most part, outside of Philadelphia. A *New York Times* article, about two and a half years after the story broke, began by stating: "Somewhere almost certainly in the United States, are as many as 70 men who could help researchers determine the risks of human exposure to the poison called dioxin."[55] The article went on to quote a clearly unre-pentant Dr. Kligman, who said: "All those people could have leukemia now—about one chance in 20 billion. And I could be hit by an asteroid when I walk out on the street, but I don't think I will."

VIII

Although the public, as well as the vast majority of inmates, allowed the dioxin story to fade from their memories, a handful of more determined and resourceful ex-prisoners turned to the legal system. In the early 1980s, several lawsuits were filed by former Holmesburg prisoners who believed they had been harmed by the Kligman-Dow experiments. If the government wouldn't redress their grievances, maybe the courts would.

Leodus Jones took his case to Common Pleas Court.[56] Jones had been an important witness at Senator Edward Kennedy's hearings in Washington a decade earlier, and had been instrumental in pressur-ing the Philadelphia prison system to terminate the medical experi-ments. "I saw the article in the *Philadelphia Tribune*[57] about the prison tests and its effects on prisoners," said Jones in a recent inter-view.[58] When he contacted the *Tribune* reporter for further informa-tion, he was "advised" to talk with an attorney.

Jones believes he was part of the dioxin experiments, and while preparing his lawsuit, "went to many hospitals [where] they did biopsies on me to see if it was." Fearing his "reproductive ability" may have been harmed by the Holmesburg tests, Jones retained legal counsel and sued Kligman, Ivy Research, the University of Pennsylvania, the prison system, and the Dow Chemical Company.

Another inmate who turned to the legal system was William Charles Smith, who had endured numerous experimental initiatives, including blister tests.[59] Smith testified that on three separate occasions a "flat, plastic device or cup containing a substance was taped to his back until it formed a blister." He said three scars remain on his back "resulting in embarrassment and emotional problems." He claimed to have sought out medical treatment in 1968 when "rashes, uncomfortable itching and cysts" appeared at the site of the original blisters.

Six years after Dow's Verald Keith Rowe revealed the controversial dioxin experiments at Holmesburg, Jones and Smith "reached out-of-court settlements with the doctor, the university, the city, and Dow Chemical Company."[60] The four defendants had challenged the allegations that Jones and Smith had taken part in the dioxin experiments, but they were unable to produce documents that conclusively showed that the former inmates didn't take part.

August Sellitto, the city's legal representative, told news reporters after the settlement that "it would be very dangerous to put this case before a jury." He said that even though the city had a minor role in the testing program, "the facts are horrible" and a "settlement seemed extremely reasonable." For Dow, the settlement represented an end to two "nuisance" suits. Gary Hamlin, a company spokesperson, said that there had been no intent to harm. "Would similar tests be performed today? Of course they wouldn't," he told inquiring reporters. Attorneys representing Smith and Jones settled out of court because they lacked sufficient documentation to prove their clients were participants in the dioxin experiments. Lawrence R. Cohan, Smith's attorney, said the deciding point came not from meeting "our burden of proof, [but] the horror factor."

The amount of the settlement was not disclosed, but Leodus Jones reports that he was awarded $40,000, a truly modest sum to such large corporate, municipal, and academic institutions. Vernon Loeb of the *Philadelphia Inquirer* searched the city records and found that the city of Philadelphia was required "to pay Smith $8,000 and Jones $5,000 as its contribution to the overall awards."[61]

If we shift the focus from the size of the individual award to the incredibly small number of plaintiffs, one asks why so few experimental subjects filed suit. When contacted by reporters after the settlement, an EPA spokesperson said that an agency search for inmates subjected to the dioxin experiments "had been able to locate only 9 inmates." According to prisoners who were interviewed, lack of knowledge and information, poor experiences with the criminal justice system, lack of money, and a false understanding of the legal ramifications of their signed waiver forms, all contributed to the passive approach taken by most of the former prison test subjects. And there was the fact that not all of the suits filed were automatic winners; some were dismissed, which left the injured party doubly wounded. James Walker, a west Philadelphia truck driver, filed suit in 1979, one year prior to Rowe's revelation about the dioxin experiment.[62] The plaintiff claimed that during two separate terms at Holmesburg in the mid-1960s, he took part in several experiments that resulted in his contracting lupus, back blisters, enlarged breasts, and a heightened sensitivity to sunlight. A year later when the dioxin experiment was revealed, Walker incorporated the Dow study in his lawsuit, which already included participation in estrogen tests and exposure to radioactive isotopes. Walker's lawyer, Albert Deutsch, said that the combination of tests ruined his client's life. "He now can work only at night, and can't enjoy his children. He can't play ball with them or go to the beach. This is hardly a normal life."[63] Deutsch described the experiments as "barbaric" and compared them to the procedures at a "Gestapo concentration camp."

James Walker and his attorney lost their case under the discovery rule, which establishes a statute of limitations on the amount of time within which a plaintiff may file suit—in Walker's case, two years. The rule states that the statute of limitations takes effect when the plaintiff knows or reasonably should have known: (1) the nature of his injury, (2) the operative cause of his injury, and (3) the causative relationship between the injury and the operative cause.

The defense argued that the clock began ticking when Walker consulted doctors at Temple University's Skin and Cancer Clinic in 1976. His two-year window of opportunity to file suit expired in

1978. Walker countered that the statute did not begin to run until he read a newspaper article, in 1979, informing him of dangerous tests at Holmesburg. The verdict of the court supported the defense. Walker, one of the very few Holmesburg human guinea pigs to file suit against Kligman and the University of Pennsylvania et al., had lost again.

Part Four

THE END OF EXPERIMENTATION AT HOLMESBURG

Seven

"Where Are We Going To Do These Things Now?"

I

The era of medical testing of Philadelphia prisoners had ended. But Solomon McBride, the longtime administrator of the human experimentation program run under the auspices of the University of Pennsylvania by Dr. Albert Kligman at Holmesburg Prison, found the termination of the once-thriving unit hard to accept. McBride was an ardent champion of the unit's work. "We weren't killing anybody," he argued emotionally to reporters covering the closure. "We haven't hurt anybody in the two decades we were there."[1]

Angered by the prison board's decision, McBride continued to plead the research unit's case. He told reporters about an additional hardship caused by the imposed closure: Ivy Research, Kligman's private research facility, which had coexisted with the University of Pennsylvania's research program, was forced to lay off 15 persons including nurses, doctors and technicians.

The January 1974 decision by the Philadelphia prison system's Board of Trustees to abolish the program came after several months of discussion and passionate debate about the merits of continuing the clinical research unit. Prison board chairman Angelo Galeone, who had repeatedly called the medical tests "demeaning and dehumanizing," was clearly relieved. "It's absolutely shut down in every respect. There is no phasing out, no completing any cycles. We're rid of it."[2]

McBride had requested additional time, a phasing-out period to give the research firm an opportunity to find new offices and new subjects for study. He expressed concern about the loss of existing and potential corporate contracts to test new products on prisoners: "We're out of business now after 20 years," said an angry McBride. "Where are we going to do these things now? Where will the new drugs come from?" He claimed the volume of business the previous year had reached $600,000, and although tests for internal drug products had already been curtailed, the consumer product testing was growing.

McBride also emphasized the program's safety and claimed the tests were harmless. He described the innocuous investigational process: "We would have a prisoner wear about five patches on his back. They would be made of tee shirt material, new cloth put out by a company. He would wear it on his back for three days and get $10. Or the patches would be a face tissue with dye on it, cosmetics, hair cream, shampoos, the stuff that goes into Brut lotion and Head and Shoulders shampoo." Not surprisingly, he did not mention that inmates had also undergone experiments using radioactive material, the carcinogenic chemical dioxin, and various psychotropic chemical warfare agents.

McBride said that the inmates benefited greatly, monetarily. In 1973, for example, 8,000 individual payments were made to inmates totaling $113,214. In addition, he said, the firm gave the city $22,642, explaining that "the system relies heavily on the use of prisoners as subjects for research." The prisoners, who without the tests had no way to earn money, closely followed the closure controversy. In fact, 750 inmates signed a petition supporting the medical testing program.

In further defense of the programs, McBride claimed: "We had one of the most advanced consent forms. We had an outside review board—a pathologist, dermatologist, minister, lawyer, sociologist—look over the programs. We're not fly-by-night. We've been taken to court I don't know how many times and it's always been dismissed." Not quite. As we have seen, the lawsuit against Kligman-Dow was setttled before it went to trial, and as we will see in this chapter, the system was at that time fending off an inmate's lawsuit asking $400,000 in damages.

Sol McBride had difficulty comprehending the board's concerns or understanding the growing criticism of human experimentation programs. As far as he and his colleagues were concerned, "to ban medical experiments completely [was] sheer folly."[3] For prison administrators, however, the research program, whether under the guise of the University of Pennsylvania or Ivy Research, was a luxury they could no longer afford. For years they had supported the program because they thought it provided a service to society by supplying the raw material—humans—for the many clinical tests required to test the new drugs that advanced medicine. In return, the county penal system received favorable newspaper coverage that praised the virtues of the program and the collective contributions of the prisoners.

Gradually, however, as McBride went to court "I don't know how many times," the tone of the news articles changed, and by the late 1960s the romance of prisoner experimentation had lost most of its appeal. Dr. Albert Kligman, himself, had generated some of the sour press, when in mid-1966 he was temporarily banned from any further experimentation by the FDA, and headlines such as "Kligman Admits Inaccuracy in Science Reporting," appeared.[4] The respected dermatologist and his prison practice were no longer immune to criticism. After the mid-1960s, the stories became skeptical and even alarming. The special prison investigation by Alan Davis, chief assistant district attorney of Philadelphia, was such a story.[5]

II

In the summer of 1968, Joseph Mitchell, then 19, and George DiAngelo, 21, two slightly built inmates, claimed they had been repeatedly raped in the prison and in sheriff's vans that transported prisoners to City Hall. Disturbed by the allegations, Judge Alexander F. Barbieri appointed District Attorney Arlen Specter's top assistant, Alan Davis, to vigorously pursue the allegations. Police Commissioner Frank L. Rizzo, never one to take a back seat when a high-profile public-safety issue was breaking, started a parallel investigation, and soon these two investigations were merged. Davis and his staff closely examined the period between June 1966 and July 1968 and interviewed more than 3,300 of the 60,000 inmates who had passed through the three-prison system during that time. They also interviewed 561 out of 570 custodial employees. After an extensive investigation that included scores of polygraph tests, the investigators "found that sexual assaults in the Philadelphia prison system [were] epidemic."[6] Further,

> As Superintendent Hendrick and three of the wardens admitted, virtually every slightly built young man committed by the courts is sexually approached within a day or two after his admission to prison. Many of these young men are repeatedly raped by gangs of inmates. Others, because of the threat of gang rape, seek protection by entering into a homosexual relationship with an individual tormentor. Only the tougher and more hardened young men, and those few so obviously frail that they are immediately locked up for their own protection, escape homosexual rape.[7]

The report graphically described how victims were targeted for sexual assault, how the attacks were carried out, and how repeated episodes of such criminal behavior went undetected and undeterred. During the 26-month period under investigation, 156 sexual assaults were documented, of which 149 occurred in the prisons and 7 in the sheriff's vans. The report estimated that when all sources of information were evaluated, "the true number of assaults...was actually about 2,000."[8]

The report then takes an ominous turn, focusing attention on the University of Pennsylvania's research testing facility at Holmesburg Prison. The connection arose from the finding that "a person with economic advantage in prison often uses it to gain sexual advantage."[9] Predatory veteran inmates, after a few days of giving cigarettes, candy, and other items to a new inmate, "will demand sexual repayment." The report described the prison economy as exceptionally bleak: "a shopworker earns 15 to 25 cents a day; half of the inmates have no prison jobs at all and most inmates get little or no material help from friends or relatives outside the prison."

Davis and his investigative colleagues said it was "the duty of prison officials to reduce the economic power that any inmate might exercise over another inmate," but there was "one area in which Philadelphia prison officials, either through neglect or indifference, disregarded this duty." The Davis report named the "large laboratory on H Block" operated by the University of Pennsylvania and a "private concern" as having a horrific effect upon daily life in the prison.

Davis went into some depth describing the facility as one set up to "test inmates' reactions to new medicines and experimental commercial products like soaps, shaving creams, suntan lotions and toilet tissue." Prisoners were viewed as "excellent human guinea pigs (1) because they live under controlled conditions, and (2) because they will submit to tests for a fraction of the fee that a free individual would demand." The report claims that "because there is very little other activity for the prisoners, and because the laboratory pays 20 percent of the inmates' wages to the prison system" the "prison officials ...have allowed the project to expand to the extent that it constitutes a separate government within the prison system." The report said:

> All of the inmates at Holmesburg wanted to "get on the tests" because, by prison standards, they can earn a fortune. Just by wearing a chemical patch on his back, for example, a prisoner can earn $10 to $15 a week. By participating in some tests that last longer, a prisoner—for doing almost nothing—will receive over $100. Altogether, the Holmesburg inmates earn more than $250,000 a year from the project. A few prisoners end up with bodies crazyquilted with motley scars and skin patches, but to these men, in the context of a prison economy, it seems well worth it.[10]

Davis reported that "to save money, the operators of the project use inmates as laboratory assistants." A prisoner could earn $100 a month for this work, which in "the prison economy, [is] the equivalent of a millionaire's income." The report concluded that "the U of P project has had a disastrous effect upon the operations of Holmesburg Prison" and stood as the critical reason "why morale of the employees is at the lowest in that institution." "The disproportionate wealth and power in the hands of a few inmates leads to favoritism, bribery, and jealousy among the guards, resulting in disrespect for supervisory authority and prison regulations." Furthermore, the university research program "contributed to homosexuality in the prison."

The report cites Stanley Randle, a 38-year-old con man serving a 4-to-11-year sentence for passing bad checks, as a particularly egregious example of the sexual abuses at Holmesburg. Housed on H Block, he was employed as a research assistant and was granted the "power to decide which inmates would serve as subjects on various tests," an extraordinarily authoritarian position for any prisoner to hold. His cell became the centerpiece of a sex-for-money scheme that paid a total of between $10,000 and $20,000 a year. In the assistant district attorney Davis's opinion, "Randle's power was considerable."

The resourceful inmate's game plan was quite simple. His "special taste was newly admitted young inmates" and through his influence with "the guard staff" he was able to pick any of them he desired as "cell mates...for as long as he wished." As soon as a new cell mate moved in, Randle "solicited them to engage in sexual acts in return for his giving them a steady stream of luxuries and for 'getting them on the tests.'" At least a half dozen individuals submitted to his lucrative experiments-for-sex arrangement. They profited "handsomely" with funds indirectly supplied by the University of Pennsylvania research project.

When confronted with the information, top prison officials were caught off balance. They told investigating officials that "no inmate was permitted to earn more than $1,200 a year," and that $400 was an "unusually high" sum for an inmate to earn as a test volunteer; but Randle's present cell mate had already earned more than $800 in just six months. According to prison records, a prior cell mate had made more than $1,700 in less than a year. Davis reported that, "When we asked university project managers about these high incomes, they told us they never heard of any $1,200 a year limit." It appeared that prison officials not only didn't know what was happening within the prison walls, but they did not control the institution. Guards who saw the activity and knew of various inmate scams claimed they "had been instructed by 'higher-ups' not to interfere in the affairs of inmates working for the U of P."[11]

Culminating months of speculation, the Davis report covered the depth and scope of corruption in the local penal system. Newspapers printed salacious details in numerous articles with attention-grabbing headlines such as "Lab Testing Program Tied to Prison Sex Corruption." Dr. Kligman called it "vile" to associate his research with homosexual abuses and argued that the Holmesburg medical lab was "closely supervised."[12] City Controller Paul M. Chalfin disagreed. He "recommended that medical testing programs on inmates at Holmesburg Prison be carried out under the guidelines of a formal contract to establish legal responsibility."[13] Although the program had been underway for 15 years, he said a contract was necessary "for the protection of the city and the inmates...should consequences ever result from the programs." It was reported that both Kligman and Superintendent Hendrick agreed with the idea of a contract, but the impact of yet another negative news story about the human research program was noticeable.

In later years, Paul Chalfin would serve on the bench as a Common Pleas Court Judge and much later as a prison board member. In an interview, Judge Chalfin said that he never truly established "why the testing program was given out to [Dr. Kligman]."[14] It had never been made clear to him "why [Kligman] was doing the tests and for whom?"

The prison system's Board of Trustees was slow to pick up on the significance of the publicity. Judge Charles Mirarchi, a board member between 1968 and 1971, says the research program was thought to be a "neutral to positive" thing, but admits "we didn't know much about it."[15] He says they were "told the tests were not dangerous" and Hendrick gave it his personal "okay." In Mirarchi's opinion, although the inmates reportedly "liked" the program, they were "not getting enough money for the tests." The prison board became, he said, "concerned about lawsuits...and the impact to the city."

Artis Ray, another prison board member during the same period, says, "I don't recall the issue of approval for testing ever coming before the board."[16] For Ray, that was just fine, since he believes "medical things should be decided by medically trained individuals. As a layman I could not determine such things." Ray says he knew little about the testing except that the program was not supposed to be "testing anything that was dangerous," and it was a "source of income for the prisoners." In his advice to the board, Superintendent Hendrick may have been trying to reassure the members about the quality of the medical research program, but his strategy was destined to fail.

III

City officials and prison board members received another embarrassing jolt when the local penal system was unfavorably highlighted in a 1973 Congressional Hearing on Human Experimentation.[17] Ostensibly designed to hear testimony about providing enhanced training on the ethical and legal implications of advances in bioethical research, the forum was really intended to address issues related to shocking revelations about the Tuskegee Syphilis Study. The lengthy and much publicized hearings became a broadside against the use of vulnerable populations—including prisoners—as medical human guinea pigs, and were a public relations disaster for those, especially the pharmaceutical industry, who supported the then-current clinical research practices.

Several influential lawyers, doctors, and authors (including Jessica Mitford, whose controversial book *Kind and Usual Punishment* had just been released) testified before the Subcommittee on Health of the Committee on Labor and Public Welfare, but the only test subjects to address the senators were two former prisoners from Philadelphia, Allan Lawson and Leodus Jones. Senator Edward Kennedy, the subcommittee chairman, was particularly impressed by the prisoners' testimony and held a lengthy dialogue with each of them.

Allan Lawson began the inmates' prepared remarks by describing the city prison system and the reasons inmates were attracted to the medical experiments. He said that 84.4 percent of the prisoners were detentioners: untried defendants waiting, on average, 9 months for a court date. "Almost all wait in idleness" because of lack of work. The few jobs that are available in prison pay "no more than 50 cents per day."[18] "This lack of jobs and the prison's failure to provide basic necessities makes the prisoners' need for money acute," said Lawson. This economic factor was critical to understanding the engine that drove the prison research program.

Perplexed, Senator Kennedy asked Lawson, "Why do you need any income in prison?"

Lawson replied, "You need it especially when you are first arrested. You have to take care of your basic necessities. You have to get an attorney. You have to try to get money together for your family.

Usually when poor guys are locked up, they are snatched off the street. If they own anything, they are going to lose it. You have to have money to protect your own belongings. The guys in prison don't have the money to make their bail...."

"Do you need any money in prison, itself?" asked Kennedy.

Lawson replied with a litany of wants and needs including tooth-paste, toothbrush, facecloths, soap, deodorant, letter-writing materials, and attorneys "to try and get your bail." He then returned to his prepared remarks and said the economic situation was so bad that a Philadelphia court had concluded that "Substantially, the only way in which a prisoner can earn money is by participation in the medical testing program conducted in the prisons by the University of Pennsylvania and Ivy Research Laboratory."[19] Lawson then launched into a closer examination of the Philadelphia medical research unit by stating that the "degrading conditions" in the jail resulted in the "trading of human bodies for money" and made "any claim of voluntary participation by prisoners in human experimentation a cruel hoax."

He followed with a brief description of Dr. Kligman's experiments and paid particular attention to experiments in the service of "private industry,...the U.S. Department of Defense, and...Dr. Kligman's personal brainstorming." Lawson described a 1971 staph infection study that involved 150 prisoners from 25 to 40 years of age, "most of whom were black." The men were infected with a staph infection and 3 became ill. Many others required antibiotic treatment, "especially those from whom skin biopsies were taken." According to Lawson, Dr. Kligman's final report stated that "on the whole, the discomfort caused by the lesions was cheerfully borne by the volunteers."[20] Another experiment called for 20 prisoners to have Johnson & Johnson baby shampoo dropped into their eyes over a 24-hour period. The discomfort of such an experience was worth $3 to each man.

At this point, Senator Kennedy inquired about the use of informed consent waivers. Lawson replied that "to most of the men in a penitentiary," reading such a document "is like reading hieroglyphics."

After describing other experiments, Lawson proceeded to mention Dr. Kligman's sanction by the FDA in 1966, and the 1968 district attorney's negative report on the relationship between prison operations and the medical research operation. Still, Lawson lamented, the experimentation program survived these controversies. To deflect criticism of the experiments, Kligman had created an institutional review board that was chaired by Dr. Howard M. Rawnsley, a University of Pennsylvania Medical School colleague. Rawnsley, according to Lawson, received "at least partial payment from the Inmates Welfare Fund for his services."[21] Another "colleague and co-author [Dr. Henry C. Maguire] of Dr. Kligman's at the university" was also on the committee. "Since last summer," said Lawson, "this committee has considered and approved approximately 80 protocols without holding any meetings. These protocols are circulated by mail and are totally inadequate for this purpose."

Lawson also claimed that inmates selected to participate in certain experiments were given "superficial and sometimes completely falsified" information. After an inmate is approved he is asked to sign the voluntary consent and financial liability waiver forms. Lawson said that since the test itself "is usually, if not always, administered by either another inmate or by a 'free world' laboratory technician...the prisoners generally do not know the nature of the test in which they are participating."

The Federal Food, Drug, and Cosmetics Act, he argued, let the experimenters off the hook; they were never held financially responsible for their acts. Even additional safeguards, such as "review committees, fully informed consent, and the highest ethical conduct are no protection if unlucky prisoners suffer present or future side effects and receive no compensation. We sincerely believe that all testing should be stopped." Lawson admitted that complete cessation of the experiments "would cut off the only present means of survival for most prisoners," but he concluded: "This is a vicious, vicious circle. Are there no 'acceptable' solutions?"

Kennedy then turned to Leodus Jones and asked him to comment on the experiments in which he had participated.

Jones said, "The only way I seen that I was able to raise bail money...was to submit to medical testing. So, I had to consider taking a chance on the testing. On one of the tests, I was told it was penicillin. The individual who told me didn't know whether it was penicillin or not. This is something he told me to get around being questioned."[22]

After Jones explained that he received $30 for taking some pills and lying "in a metabolic ward for about two nights," Kennedy returned to an issue he was still troubled by, the need for money in prison. "Do the people that have money in prison, are they able to control their environment? Is it a better life if they have money in prison?"

"Yes," said Jones, the money made a world of difference.

"Did the guards treat you differently if you had money?" asked Kennedy.

"Generally, they treat you differently," Jones responded. "I think in most situations, whether it is in a penitentiary or in the street, if you have money, you are better off."

Kennedy then turned to the possibility of an inmate's withdrawing from a test after the experiment was underway. Jones said they could, but such a decision was not without consequences. He told of men in one test who had "these germs" placed on their arms, backs, and legs, but after the test was over and they were released from prison, they didn't know what to do "if they [broke] out in a rash." He told the committee that he had been on one test where "some type of germ from India" was placed on his arm. After five days an infection set in and his arm began to swell, but he was released from prison before the experiment was over and the wound had not completely healed. He expressed concern about whether the substance applied to his arm would affect him in the future. "These people go into it blind," Jones argued. "They don't know nothing about nothing. Those who conduct the tests don't know nothing about nothing. These are just experiments."

Senator Kennedy inquired about general prison conditions, including the plight of untried detentioners and the overall hygiene in the prisons. After hearing a bleak description of "four guys jammed in a cell...damp air...no hot water" and several other conditions contributing to the Philadelphia prison system being declared "cruel and unusual punishment," Kennedy asked Lawson and Jones if the opportunity "to get out of those cells" and try some experimental drugs "sounded pretty good?"[23]

Lawson replied firmly that the offer of money was the key attraction. "Generally," he said, "you could volunteer for an hour's work around the penitentiary to get out of the cell, but you don't get paid there. The only job they have available will pay you 50 cents. It is more...the money than just [getting] out of the cell."

The appearance of the former Holmesburg inmates at high-profile Senate hearings in Washington distressed the Philadelphia Prison board and other city officials. Not only was the penal system revealed to be engaged in a practice that was frowned on nationally, but these revelations were also well publicized. Congressional investigations illuminated slipshod medical practices, improper informed consent procedures, and dangerous experiments that took advantage of an ignorant, destitute, and vulnerable population. The human experimentation program had to be terminated.

Jones and Lawson were proud to have gone to Washington, to have testified before a full Senate committee and taken a stand against a shoddy medical practice, but the reaction from the prisoners whose cause they championed was anger. "Leodus and I was happy when the tests were stopped, but we were cussed out when we were back up at the jail," said Lawson when I interviewed him.[24] "They wrote us letters about that stuff. They really wanted the money." Two decades after the experiments were concluded, Lawson and Jones still wince when recounting the reaction of fellow inmates.

For two prisoners to risk the pressure of their peers, to so influence a program's closure—and to have gained such national exposure—is a testament to their characters and political sophistication. Lawson had gone into prison with a skill; he knew the law, or enough of it to pass as a decent jailhouse lawyer. Through his mastery of the legal process, Lawson was able to earn money and avoid the experiments on H Block. "I found a new way to get out of jail without dying or going over the wall," he says. "If you were a petition writer, you were a big man in the jail. I learned it from the best writers in the jail."

It was probably because of Lawson's legal reputation in the jail that several inmates sought him out about the University of Pennsylvania research unit. "Guys in prison asked us to investigate the prison experimentation program," he recalls. Although a majority of the men had no complaints about the experiments, a few were concerned and wanted the testing project ended. He says that people were more "politicized" in those days; African-American inmates were particularly fearful of "genocide" and suspected that black prisoners were recruited for the more dangerous experiments. Lawson and his fellow inmates began to investigate the program and "put together a coalition of groups [on the outside] that had fragments and pieces" of useful information. The Philadelphia Yearly Meeting of the Religious Society of Friends, Community Legal Services, the Barbwire Society, and a number of churches and community groups, among other organizations, began to monitor human research practices at Holmesburg Prison. Typical was a small community group called Degrees of Captivity, founded by a nurse, Mattie Humphrey, who was "appalled" by what she felt was the "illegal use of prisoners for research purposes."[25] She believed the research was a "serious, gross problem" that "made money for the pharmaceutical companies" and typified the general "attitude that African-Americans were subhuman" and "everything bad [could be] targeted toward" them.

Lawson and Jones approached the American Civil Liberties Union. "The Philadelphia chapter of the ACLU was concerned with medical testing of inmates at Holmesburg," says Spencer Coxe, longtime executive director of the organization.[26] "The prisoners were in a coercive position....[They] needed money and testing was it." But, recalls Coxe, since it was a "source of income" for the financially destitute prisoners, the ACLU did not take the position of "all-out opposition to prisoner testing." He says that "an all-out position was my own view, but Allan Lawson argued against it." In addition, some members of the ACLU believed that the organization should not arbitrarily tell people how to live their lives. Coxe is still troubled by his organization's halfhearted position on prison experimentation. "In retrospect it was a mistake," says Coxe. "It was an honest and understandable position. It was defensible, but wrong in retrospect."

At state government hearings in Harrisburg, three months after Senator Kennedy's hearings, prisoners' rights attorney David Rudovsky presented the formal ACLU position on prison medical experimentation. The organization offered the following guidelines:

1. All consents obtained for the purposes of any form of experimentation must be informed consents.

2. It is the responsibility of the researcher to make sure that the prospective volunteer is in the proper physical and (when relevant) mental condition to undertake the experiment.

3. Waiver forms or exculpatory language in the consent document must be banned.

4. Researchers must be required to carry insurance providing total coverage for subjects adversely affected by the experiment, and for compensation of the family or next of kin in case of death.

5. Prisoner-volunteers must be paid at a scale commensurate with what the researcher would offer "free world" volunteers as compensation.

6. Prisoners should not be promised reduced sentences or favorable consideration for parole in return for participation in a clinical experiment.

7. Assurances must be made and enforced that the experiment will be carried out in a manner that does not necessarily threaten the lives or safety of the prisoner-volunteers.

8. Subject to requirement number 6, no report or records of the prisoners' participation in the experiments should be released to anyone by the researcher or by prison authorities without the signed consent of the prisoners.

9. A supervisory committee, independent of prison authorities, the researcher, and the sponsors of the research, must be established to review and oversee all experimentation conducted in prisons.

10. The sponsors of prison research (drug companies, foundations, or whoever) must pay reasonable sums for the privilege of having access to the inmate population for research purposes.

11. Prison authorities should immediately undertake to provide greater opportunities for prisoners to work and earn money.[27]

Rudovsky concluded his statement by stressing that "guidelines represent the minimum conditions and safeguards" for prisoner experimentation. If those could not be achieved, then a "moratorium on experimentation in prisons should be extended indefinitely."

The coalition that formed to fight prison medical testing in Philadelphia was far from a political juggernaut representing a cross-section of the city's religious, labor, and civic groups. Organizations one would expect to be part of such an effort were either not involved or late in joining the campaign. Probably the best example of this was the Pennsylvania Prison Society, the nation's oldest prison reform organization dating back to 1787. "It was never an issue that came before the board," says Marvin Wolfgang, a highly respected criminologist at the University of Pennsylvania and Prison Society president during most of the 1960s.[28] "Kligman was doing tests almost clandestinely, secretively. We knew very little about it," Wolfgang says. "The experiments were thought to have a public health benefit. There were no complaints and the inmates presumably were volunteers." Professor Wolfgang says the "widespread use of prisoners" as research subjects in postwar America was commonplace and therefore unalarming. This attitude, especially from a prison watchdog organization, symbolized the general public's acceptance of such medical practices that had helped to foster human experimentation in prisons for many years. But by the early 1970s, the tide had turned; community and professional opposition was building, and the legal repercussions were beginning to take their toll.

IV

The first significant legal problem regarding human research at Holmesburg arose when 9 black, male "subjects" between the ages of 23 and 31 years of age volunteered to test the safety and tolerance of W-2429, a new medication developed by Wallace Laboratories. One of the nine was Jerome Roach, a detainee awaiting trial, who decided to "participate because he needed money to pay for minimal needs and comforts" while incarcerated. "After four days of taking temperature pills," Roach developed "various symptoms of physical illness including sore throat, sore joints, fever, nausea and sores and rashes."[29] In addition, Roach complained that he received improper treatment from the prison physician, "who prescribed penicillin without knowing or inquiring if Roach was participating in an experiment." By March 29, 1973, Roach's condition had grown serious enough for him to be transferred to Philadelphia General Hospital, where he remained for several weeks. Roach claimed that at the hospital, he was told his illness "resulted from the experiment and he had been given pills different from those described to him when he consented to the experiment, and that he had permanent liver damage."

Furthermore, Roach argued, his condition grew worse when he returned to his prison cell after leaving the hospital. Kept in a cold, wet cell and denied adequate medical treatment and medication for two weeks in June 1973, Roach believed his civil rights had been violated. He retained legal counsel and sued Dr. Kligman, Ivy Research Laboratories, the prison system, and the city for $400,000.[30] His attorney was David Rudovsky, a young lawyer who had already developed a keen interest in prison reform issues (he'd presented findings for the ACLU to the Pennsylvania Department of Justice & Public Welfare just 3 years earlier) and had just embarked on what would become a quarter century of litigation against the city for its poor management of the county jail.

According to Rudovsky's recollection, Roach was "never specifically informed of what he was being exposed to, [or] any adverse reactions" that might have occurred.[31] Furthermore, he had been the victim of "bad aftercare"; the consent forms inmate-volunteers were made to sign were "not legitimate"; and Kligman's program could best be characterized as following generally "sloppy methods of research."

The depositions Rudovsky took from Dr. Kligman and his associates are interesting for the specifics of the Roach case, as well as for the light they shed on the overall operations of the Holmesburg research program. Dr. Kligman asserted that the "monetary savings" of using prisoners over "free world" volunteers was secondary to the fact that "the prisons provided total control of the test population."[32] And although "events of this kind [the lawsuit] make us very nervous," said Kligman, Roach's reaction to W-2429, "a mild analgesic," may have been due to his "receiving shots of penicillin by prison doctors [physicians unrelated to the human research program] who were unaware Roach was on a test."

Herbert Copelan, the key physician for the research program, who specialized in internal medicine, testified that "Roach had no allergic reaction to the drug" used in the experiment.[33] Although doctors at Philadelphia General Hospital "thought Roach had mononucleosis," Copelan thought he "had serum sickness." In addition, Copelan said it was not his job to "warn or brief" prisoners prior to their participation in the tests—that was done by Luther Mitchell. A licensed practical nurse, Mitchell said he told volunteers "what the tests [were] about," but "did not explain what side effects [there] would be. That," he said, "was Dr. Copelan's area."[34]

The depositions revealed additional information about the development of inmate consent forms, the informal agreements between Kligman and Superintendent Hendrick, and the roles various individuals played in the testing program.

As was commonplace in many prison research programs in the 1950s, Kligman's program "at first...had no consent forms, [but] became more and more formalized as [it] went along."[35] The one-page consent form used in the "Safety and Tolerance of W-2429" study was probably typical of those used in the last years of the Holmesburg research operation. Under the title "Consent to Participate in Medical Study," the inmate-volunteers were asked to sign a document that spelled out the participants' understanding that "the study may involve some hazard or discomfort and some unknown risk or result," that the individual "freely volunteered for the test without any force, pressure or inducement other than payment," and "that neither the Philadelphia Prisons nor the City of Philadelphia are [sic] responsible for any undesirable effects that may occur because of the study, and I agree that I shall make no claim against them." The document concluded with: "In consideration of the sum of $1.00 I hereby accept any risks of this study and release Dr. H. W. Copelan, M.D., his assistants and Ivy Research Laboratories, Inc. for any action or claim for injury or illness which may occur because of my participation."[36]

Kligman testified that the "inmate studies had two purposes: (1) commercial studies for profit and (2) medical research with no commercial implications."[37] On the subject of a formal arrangement with the city, he said, "There never was a contract with the city....it was an ad hoc sort of arrangement. As we went along, we developed more and more interchange with the city officials, but there never was a legal document authorizing our exercise." Many years of prisoner experimentation had been founded on "an oral agreement with the superintendent." [It is interesting to note here that in the early- and mid-1950s, Dr. Norman R. Ingraham, Jr., was the deputy public

health commissioner of Philadelphia at the same time that he held
the position of assistant professor and budget administrator of the
University of Pennsylvania's dermatology department.[38] In short, Dr.
Ingraham as a university administrator oversaw payments to Dr.
Kligman and other university personnel, and as a city official over-
saw the establishment of county-wide health policy.]

Asked by Rudovsky about "money for rent, or payment for use of
the facilities?" Kligman responded, "Yes, there was a fixed fee....I
think it was 20 percent of whatever the prisoners were paid."
Rudovsky verified: "So that means if you had ten prisoners in the
test, each getting one hundred dollars, which would be a thousand?
You would also pay..."

"The prison would get two hundred," was Kligman's ready reply.

Asked if "there were other arrangements for payment to the city
for the use of the facilities," Kligman said, "I don't think so."

Monies accumulated did not stay in the prison system, however.
According to Jack Hepp, Jr., who handled the inmates' accounts as
well as the prison system's financial records, "the money was sent
to the city treasury."[39] Hepp, who started working for the prison system in 1959, says "the experiments were in full swing" by the time
of his arrival and he doesn't remember seeing "a formal contract at
any time." The paperwork for inmate accounts kept him quite busy.
"We would get checks from Ivy and Clover Labs [Kligman private
companies] on a weekly basis. The inmates got the money...for various experiments...like flu studies and other tests. It would be a dollar or two a piece on some studies" and considerably more on others.
He "put the money on the books" (the inmates' prison accounts), but
"took it off" almost as quickly because the prisoners immediately
"spent it on commissary items....The paperwork for those experiments and the payments to the inmates was quite a job [because]
huge numbers of inmates were involved."

Hepp now claims to have had "mixed feelings" about the testing
program. "Inmates participated because they were broke and needed
the money. When you're in a desperate situation you do things you
might not ordinarily do....There were risks involved that otherwise
they would not have taken. I thought it was good initially, but later
revelations came out about other tests" that were quite disturbing.

V

Rudovsky queried Ivy and prison officials about their research program's institutional review board (IRB). Starting in the late 1960s and building momentum by the early 1970s, federal agencies had begun encouraging additional institutional protections for research subjects. "The rights and welfare of subjects...informed consent, and the balance of risks and benefits" were the dominant interests of the newly emerging IRBs.[40]

Throughout the *Roach v. Kligman* legal proceedings, both Ivy and prison officials used the IRB to bolster their defense and demonstrate the "innocuous" nature of the experiments that were initiated at Holmesburg. Referring to the establishment of an IRB at the prisons in the early 1970s (no doubt encouraged by the requirements of the overseers for the Army experiments), Kligman said in his deposition that "the thrust of the times required it. The prison was getting, you know, in the absence of a contract, they wanted some defense, they wanted to feel more stable in what we were doing, and so did we. This gave us...an official way to recognize what we were doing."[41]

Superintendent Louis G. Aytch, Hendrick's successor in 1971, concurred. "All clinical investigation," Aytch said, "is conducted under the guidelines of the United States Food and Drug Administration, The United States Department of Health, Education and Welfare (National Institutes of Health Protection of Human Subjects Policies and Procedures), The American Correctional Association, the Declaration of Helsinki...and the Nuremberg Code."[42] Aytch said that "the committee includes an attorney, clergyman, sociologist and two more physicians experienced in medical research. No project may be authorized unless every member of the panel independently gives approval."

The IRB became a very convenient shield against those who attacked the prison research program or questioned aspects of the experiments. David Rudovsky did not have the opportunity to question the IRB panel members, but in recent interviews they talked about what they remembered of board activity.

The IRB's chairman, Dr. Howard M. Rawnsley, says that the committee members received a regular stipend for their participation.

Then a board-certified pathologist and the director of the William Pepper Laboratory at the University of Pennsylvania Hospital, Rawnsley says "each protocol brought a $5 fee. About 20 to 30 protocols would come in batches and the checks would come from Ivy Research."[43] Dr. Rawnsley "couldn't remember the number of times" that the committee met, but he does recall "one tour of Holmesburg."

Henry C. Maguire, the other physician on the Holmesburg IRB, was no stranger to either Dr. Kligman or the research experiments at the county jail. Maguire, in fact, had trained under Kligman in the University of Pennsylvania's dermatology department and had published several journal articles with his mentor in the early 1960s.[44] Maguire said he spent about "three or four years" on the committee, but "it was not that active a group." In fact, he said "I can't remember we ever met. There were no formal meetings."[45]

The attorney on the panel was Seymour M. Johnson, Jr., an acquaintance of Superintendent Aytch. Johnson recalls little of his association with the prison IRB, but says "I wouldn't know anything about the medical stuff. I relied on them [the doctors] for the decision."[46]

The sociologist on the panel was Cecil O. Smith, Jr., the acting chairman of Drexel University's social science department. Smith recalls being asked to join the newly formed peer review committee by Dr. Rawnsley, a neighbor who was active with Smith on the neighborhood townwatch group. "The committee was set up to deflect criticism," says Smith.[47] There was "no review committee prior to the new federal regulations, and one needed to be established. They needed nonmedical people [and] the regulation [specified] a social scientist." Smith remembers that the "protocols came in large envelopes...[they were] quite thick and didn't make too much sense to a layman....The dermatologist [Dr. Maguire] would explain what the test was....The lay members did not really know what was going on."

Despite their medical ignorance, Smith believes that the committee was serious and hoped to ward off negative public opinion. He remembers the dermatologic patch tests only, and believes that any experiments using "hallucinogens would have been rejected." Smith also recalls that their payment as board members became an issue. He says they were initially paid about $1,000 a year, but payment was terminated after the "Unitarian minister" expressed his concern about receiving payment for tests to which he had an obligation to remain neutral.

The minister in question was Rev. Victor H. Carpenter of the First Unitarian Church in Center City Philadelphia. He clearly recalls what eventually became a very troubling association. He says Dr. Rawnsley, whom he did not know at the time, "came to my church one Sunday and asked if I would serve on this prison committee."[48] Carpenter thought his participation would be a beneficial, humanitarian gesture and accepted. He remembers, however, that he quickly became disillusioned. He began to receive the protocols in the mail, but there were no meetings. For two years, "[he] never met another member" of the committee. Carpenter says he "became increasingly uncomfortable" and requested a meeting. He became more uncomfortable still when he started to receive money for what he thought was voluntary service. "The checks started to arrive….several hundred dollars. I was surprised….The whole issue became disturbing….There was a total lack of supervision of the protocols and the process. We were left to our own devices with no guidance or direction. When the checks arrived it really raised my suspicions." He asked Dr. Rawnsley about the money and was told that it was "simply gratitude from the pharmaceutical companies." Rev. Carpenter says that the situation became so disquieting that he "returned the last check…and wrote a letter expressing my concerns and submitting my resignation from the board." The minister was so troubled by his association with the prison system's review board that he went to Harrisburg and testified at legislative hearings on human experimentation abuses in the state's penal institutions. Brought in as a protector, his exposure to the human research program made him an opponent.

VI

During the last few years of the Holmesburg research program, state authorities were taking an increasingly skeptical look at prison drug testing operations throughout Pennsylvania. The state prison system held no experimental drug testing units, but a small number of counties still allowed these research units in their local jails. "We had little overall influence," says Allyn Sielaff, the commissioner of corrections for the state of Pennsylvania from 1968 to 1973, "but we tried to strengthen our inspections" of county facilities.[49] Currently a criminal justice professor at a small liberal arts college in northwest Pennsylvania, Sielaff says he has long been opposed to such medical programs and "avoided [them] scrupulously." He believes an experimental research program, like the one in Holmesburg, was successful because it offered the only opportunity for inmates to earn money. But, he continues, "I would hardly call it [the choice to participate in experiments] voluntary. The prisoners should have other [ways] to make money for it to be voluntary. If it were truly voluntary, an inmate could say, 'Instead of working in the metal shop I'd like to get bit by a tsetse fly.' But since there is no other real way to make money in prison, [the inmate cannot make] a voluntary decision."

Finally, one of those most concerned about prison issues was newly elected state legislator Lucien Blackwell. "As soon as I got to Harrisburg in 1972...I got involved in the issue," recalls the former U. S. congressman in an interview.[50] Blackwell says he "was new to politics" back then and just learning the ropes of elected public service, but when he started to receive numerous phone calls from constituents about conditions at Holmesburg Prison, he felt he had to pay attention to prison issues. After conferring with David Richardson, another interested African-American legislator from Philadelphia, Blackwell set up an official tour for members of the recently formed Legislative Black Caucus.

"The guards gave us a hard time," says Blackwell. "They didn't want us there. They really were not too helpful." Still, the lawmakers toured the cell blocks and talked to the prisoners. "The inmates were being treated rather poorly," Blackwell recalls. "Old men 75 years old were sharing the same cell as teenagers, the food was terrible, and the medical care less than adequate."

When the visitors asked about the medical testing program, they met strong and divided opinions. "Some inmates were offended by the program and others wanted to keep it." Blackwell says he talked to one inmate-participant in a study in which a new drug was being dropped into his eyes. It looked quite uncomfortable. "Why would you risk injuring your eyes?" Blackwell asked him. The inmate's answer was the same as that from all the other prisoners they heard—money. Some of the inmates were upset that Blackwell and his colleagues were challenging the existence of the research program. "[They said] 'You're hurting us. We want the tests. They don't give you soap or a comb if you need it because you're going to court.' With money from the tests they could buy those things...and send...money home to their wives and children."

Despite those pleas, Blackwell came to believe that the medical experiments were dangerous and took advantage of the inmates. He introduced legislation to end all such experimentation in Pennsylvania prisons. To his surprise, "about a month or two after I had introduced the bill," Milton Shapp, the newly elected governor, issued an executive order ending medical testing in prisons. "He stole my thunder and issue, and never even called me," said Blackwell, but it was done.

Eight

"Retin-A®'s Birthplace Was at Holmesburg Prison."

I

The advertisements for Renova®, the latest youth enhancer—that promises to dwarf in sales and fame Retin-A, its popular predecessor—are bold, no-nonsense, and attention-grabbing. Despite a flock of commercial imitators, Renova's advertising as "the only prescription cream proven to treat fine wrinkles" carries the aura of scientific credibility.[1] No expense has been spared to promote the "specially designed and patented water-in-oil emulsion." Magazine and journal advertisements for the much discussed product are rarely limited to one page; three-page promotions have become standard. And dermatologists, a critical target of the advertising blitz, have been bombarded with generous five-page buys in *Archives of Dermatology*, a journal widely read in the profession.

The product behind this high-powered Madison Avenue artistry is an Ortho Pharmaceutical facial elixir that is said to do wonders with fine wrinkles, brown spots, and rough skin. Renova®, a gentler repackaging of Retin-A® (retinoid acid), the vitamin A derivative used since the early 1970s to combat acne, has become the most-talked-about "fountain of youth in a tube" throughout the cosmetic industry, and a wellspring of corporate profit. The .05 percent tretinoin emollient cream, on which the FDA delayed approval for six turbulent years, eventually drew the wrath of the U.S. attorney general's office. Ultimately, a staggering, multimillion-dollar fine was leveled against Ortho, a subsidiary of Johnson & Johnson. On a smaller scale, this episode made up the latest chapter in Albert M. Kligman's career as a scientist and researcher. While some may be aware of Dr. Kligman's connection to the product, few if any are aware of the critical role played by the human guinea pigs of Holmesburg Prison.

Anointed by the media as the "Father of Retin-A®" and the "Wrinkle Warrior," Dr. Kligman was not the first physician to become intrigued by the curative powers of retinoid acid, but he may have been the first to foresee its strong market appeal. Vitamin A was used by Chinese doctors more than 3,000 years ago to cure night blindness, and over the last century, retinol, retinal, and retinoic acid (vitamin A derivatives) were explored by numerous researchers as cures for a variety of ills. In the 1920s, the link "between vitamin A and cancer" was discovered "when rats fed a vitamin A–deficient diet were found to develop carcinomas of the stomach."[2]

By the 1940s dermatologists had begun to seriously examine vitamin A's potential use against acne. Jonathan V. Straumfjord "caused a great stir among dermatologists" by demonstrating that large doses of the vitamin could interrupt the embarrassing and disfiguring skin disease.[3] In one of Dr. Straumfjord's experiments that led him to believe acne may be due to vitamin A deficiency, patients with acne were treated with a supplement of approximately 100,000 international units of vitamin A daily for a minimum of six months. Seventy-nine of the patients became free from eruption and only three were unimproved.[4] Straumfjord was also one of the first to recognize that "a definite aggravation occurs in many during the early stages of treatment." He called this effect on the skin "efflorescence" and said it could last from a month or two to much longer. Subsequent experimental studies using vitamin A both topically and orally demonstrated the substance's vast potential.

Most of the vitamin A studies just prior to Dr. Kligman's research were initiated by European physicians. For those American dermatologists pursuing acne remedies, the experiments by two German physicians, Beer and Stuttgen, were landmark studies demanding replication and further experimentation. In a much-read 1962 analysis, Stuttgen wrote, "Vitamin A acid, given by mouth is efficacious as vitamin A palmitate in treating anomalies of keratinization of the skin." He cautioned that the acid has "an intense keratolytic action which is accompanied by irritation of the skin" and therefore requires a "weaker" dosage to mitigate its destructive impact.[5]

Today, Dr. Stuttgen is only mildly surprised by Retin-A®'s financial success. As a past consultant to Ortho Pharmaceutical, he had advised corporate management that retinoids would have "great application" in the future.[6] "I gave the Ortho people confidence that vitamin A acid would be a successful product," says Stuttgen. He points out that America is not alone in its fascination with the retinoid cream ("It is also successful in Europe") but he believes the European version of "vitamin A derivative is less irritable to the skin." According to Dr. Stuttgen, the irritation factor is important. He claims to have taken his vitamin A studies only so far because the "irritation of the acid was very strong" and somewhat alarming. "I was turned off by so much irritation." About Kligman's approach, he says, "irritation of the skin was a handicap he did not respect." While more conservative physicians curtailed usage, Kligman kept encouraging patients, and requiring prisoners, to continue using the medication.

Beer and Stuttgen's groundbreaking experiments would soon be overshadowed by an aggressive team of physician-researchers from the University of Pennsylvania using inmates at Holmesburg Prison as their test subjects. Apparently, Dr. Philip Frost, a resident at the Hospital of the University of Pennsylvania in the early 1960s, sparked the team's scientific interest in vitamin A. Dr. Frost recalls that he had become curious about vitamin A after he "read about its use from a couple of articles by Beer and Stuttgen."[7] He says that while the "papers...weren't terribly useful," they piqued his interest enough so that he ordered a supply of the vitamin A derivative from Switzerland. During Frost's initial applications of the drug, Kligman noticed the subject's skin reaction. "Dr. Kligman saw that [vitamin A acid] irritated the skin and asked if he could work with it," says Frost. "When I left in 1963, they had just started to use the drug on the inmates at Holmesburg."

The new dermatological irritant triggered Dr. Kligman's curiosity. The chemical was supplied free-of-charge by Hoffman-LaRoche, an international drug company based in North Jersey and Switzerland, and almost immediately Kligman assigned residents to explore the vitamin's potential. Penn Labs did the first clinical tests of what eventually would be known as Retin-A®, but the early human trials were performed on the backs and faces of the Holmesburg inmates.

As the university team tested for minimum and maximum dosage levels of different chemical compositions, the inmates suffered through the most dangerous, and certainly the most uncomfortable, phase of the clinical testing process. In a recent interview on the history of Retin-A® for *Philadelphia Magazine,* Kligman is quoted as saying that in the early stages he experimented with "very high doses" of vitamin A, so high that "I damn near killed people [before] I could see a real benefit....Everyone of them got sick."[8] Kligman was experimenting with very high dosages, sometimes orally. Eventually various derivatives of vitamin A were tried topically and the results were impressive.

"Retin-A®'s birthplace was at Holmesburg Prison," says Dr. Gerd Plewig, a resident at the University of Pennsylvania during this time, and currently chairman of the department of dermatology at the University of Munich.[9] "[The] pretesting for safety and tolerance was [conducted] at Holmesburg." Plewig, like other observers, believes Kligman's work with retinoids was his most notable achievement. "Vitamin A acid for acne treatment was his greatest success. It eventually led to systemic treatment of Retin-A® for acne."

Interestingly, the initial vitamin A experiments were targeted not at treating acne but at keratotic disorders (a thickening of the outer layer of the skin). According to the recollections of Dr. Chalmers Cornelius, also a resident during these years, an assortment of chemicals was being applied in the search for antikeratinizing agents, including sulfur and resorcinol lotions, benzoyl peroxide, and vitamin A acid. The last proved the most successful, since it caused this thick outer layer of skin to fall off, but the experiments used "much higher doses" than would be prescribed in later years.[10] These earlier studies used "1 percent vitamin A acid, in comparison to the .01 percent" adopted years later. Cornelius says some of the "occlusion studies" resulted in "tremendous inflammation and the experiments had to be altered."

Dr. Cornelius says that it was the inflammation that most attracted Kligman. Despite what many would have considered a caution sign, as in Dr. Stuttgen's reaction to the strong irritation caused by vitamin A acid, Kligman's response was always the same: "Push on." "He had that type of mentality—push on. Kligman was always pushing forward," comments Cornelius. (While this is surely an admirable trait, we need to remember that the inmates bore the brunt of Kligman's push.)

This ability to see what others couldn't, and to pursue goals from which others backed away, are the Kligman attributes that Dr. Joseph Witkowski finds so impressive. A former student of Kligman and a former director of the University of Pennsylvania's Acne Clinic, Witkowski says that he "thought [Retin-A®] would never sell. It caused a severe reaction in patients. Their faces became quite red and irritated. But Kligman has the capacity to keep pushing when others won't. He could see the value of Retin-A® as possible therapy. Time has shown that it has positive results. It's a fantastic drug. He's a genius."[11]

The doctors continued to apply retinoic acid to the faces of Holmesburg inmates and patients at the university's acne clinic. One side of the face received Retin-A® and the other side received an application of a different experimental agent, then the lesions on each side of the face were counted at weekly intervals. "The Retin-A® side always got worse before it got better," says Cornelius.

No one was more intrigued by the chemical's early test results and its dermatological potential than Albert Kligman. These were the years of the dioxin studies for Dow Chemical, the chemical warfare experiments for the Army, and the FDA investigation, but Kligman's research with vitamin A continued unabated. He assigned his dermatological residents an array of studies using the drug. Initially, Kligman believed that vitamin A acid curbed the production of old or dead skin cells, which come together, clog pores, and form a pimple. Eventually, he would reverse his thinking and argue that the vitamin actually keeps the cells apart and inhibits the formation of blackheads leading to acne.

By the late 1960s, medical journals were publishing a number of scholarly articles, written by members of the department of dermatology at the University of Pennsylvania School of Medicine, on topical vitamin A acid. In 1969, Kligman, Plewig, and James E. Fulton, Jr., published a paper that reported:

> Vitamin A acid is a fairly potent irritant. Although most acne
> remedies inflame the skin to some degree, the effects of vitamin A
> acid are rather singular. Within 48 hours the skin becomes red and

scaling. Despite prolonged usage, its irritancy does not greatly diminish; that is to say, there is only slight evidence of hardening. The skin tends to burn and sting for a short time after each application. Injudicious use may induce a flaming red, chapped, swollen face. The daily application has to be regulated in accordance with individual susceptibility. The aim is to apply that quantity which will maintain moderate redness and peeling. Discomfiture about the mouth and angles of the nose is particularly disagreeable if the medication is carelessly applied. Even with excessive use, the skin recovers within a few days after stopping treatment. Deeply motivated subjects should not be dissuaded from increasing the frequency of application for patients with the most irritated faces achieve the most rapid improvement.[12]

Kligman had already shifted his corporate allegiance from Hoffmann-LaRoche to Johnson & Johnson, with whom he had a long-time relationship and who were more interested in Retin-A®'s development. Kligman and Johnson & Johnson's joint efforts resulted in the drug coming on the market in 1971 as a treatment for severe cases of acne. And Ortho began advertising. A typical example is a glossy, two-page ad featuring Laura Shavin, an attractive 20-year-old, who declares:

> I'm pretty lucky to have a dermatologist for a dad. When my face broke out, he gave me Retin-A®. Right Away. He told me Retin-A® would clear up my acne and help keep it from coming back. My acne's gone now, and my dad says I look beautiful. Of course, he always says that. But this time, I feel beautiful, too. And as long as I'm on Retin-A®, I'm confident my acne will stay under control. After all, my dad hasn't let me down yet. Retin-A® Right Away.[13] (©Ortho Pharmaceutical Corporation)

The FDA's approval of the drug also spurred Kligman's well-developed marketing sense. Never loathe to publicize a new drug's capabilities to the public, he informed one of many newspaper reporters who did stories on the drug, "It's no cure [but the] new agent has proven to be of significant benefit in 70% to 80% of the cases studied."[14] Many of the cases studied were those of Holmesburg prisoners, and he described how they had endured "chemically induced patches of acne" in order to test the new vitamin A acid.

Brief articles also appeared illuminating the financial rewards of his pursuits. A 1970 article informed readers that the John A.

Hartford Foundation had awarded the University of Pennsylvania a three-year grant of $320,940 to study acne.[15] The hefty award followed the large Hartford grant that had led Dr. Kligman to the development of "vitamin A acid as an effective agent to treat acne."

Because of the success of Retin-A®, as well as the termination of the Holmesburg Prison research program in 1974, an increasing amount of Kligman's time was being spent on acne, retinoic acid, tretinoin, and the skin's aging. With the loss of the prison testing base and consequent loss of some of his contractual relationships, Kligman began to focus more of his attention on what he called "cosmeceuticals"—a gray but rapidly emerging area between fancy cosmetics and serious pharmaceuticals.[16]

II

Throughout the 1970s, Kligman and his associates were churning out dozens of journal articles on the medicinal affects of retinoic acid on a host of troubling skin diseases. As its most ardent champion, Kligman was loathe to believe that Retin-A® would be relegated to the narrow role of a pimple fighter. It was much more substantial than that, he believed. And potentially more profitable. Dr. Kligman claimed that for years his acne patients had been telling him Retin-A® was not only controlling their acne but making them look younger as well. At first he hadn't believed them: "I have always told students that if you start to believe your patients, you're gonna end up as a quack. So, I wasn't too smart about this....I have a doctrine: Don't believe patients. So I was a victim of my doctrine."[17]

Apparently, Kligman was won over and began to see the antiaging properties of his anti-acne cream. He had been studying what he termed photoaging, the sun's damaging effects on the skin, and began to believe that Retin-A® could reverse the impact of accumulated sun damage. Too much exposure to the sun had been known to prompt the formation of abnormal elastic fibers in the skin. Collagen underwent degeneration, dermal blood vessels dilated, and some were destroyed. This photoaging process eventually resulted in discolored, leathery, wrinkled skin, sprinkled with age spots.

In order to document Retin-A®'s anti-photoaging properties Kligman undertook a series of experiments using both animals and humans. Some of the most dramatic results occurred in mice. According to the 1979 journal publication entitled "The Effects on Rhino Mouse Skin of Agents which Influence Keratinization and Exfoliation," the impact of Retin-A® on mouse wrinkles was extraordinary.[18] Published with his third wife, Lorraine, a biochemist, Kligman chose rhino mice, an unusual species from Africa, because the mice develop rows of wrinkles from nose to rump, shortly after birth. The authors believed the wrinkle canals were filled with the same horny substance that formed pimples in humans. In their experiment, the mice received applications of Retin-A® twice a day for six weeks while a control group received none.

The results were incredible; after only three weeks the Retin-A® group had undergone a total body transformation, they were practically free of wrinkles. The skin of the control group was covered by seemingly endless wrinkles. As the Kligmans said in their conclusion: "The outstanding finding was the capacity of retinoic acid to restore the bizarre architecture of rhino mouse skin to a nearly normal appearance. [T]he treated skin became as smooth as the...hairless mouse; the redundant folds and wrinkles were totally effaced."[19] The article's startling before-and-after photographs of retinoic acid-treated mice no doubt caught the attention of the journal's readers.

In subsequent clinical trials, Retin-A® demonstrated greater blood flow and wound-healing properties along with its wrinkle-reducing powers. Kligman believed he was investigating a wonder drug with enormous scientific and financial potential. Unfortunately, the potential was dependent upon FDA approval and good product marketing, elements that were outside of the doctor's control.

Dr. Kligman, however, was not about to let his latest dermatological creation be controlled by heavy-handed government bureaucrats and deliberate corporate types. He decided to inject his own tactical ability and marketing savvy into the equation. His plan was simple: circumvent one and supply the marketing strategy for the other.

Kligman's critical gameplan was broached with an Ortho Pharmaceutical executive for the first time on January 17, 1983. (The two-page interoffice memo of that momentous meeting would become a key part of the federal government's case against the drug company years later.) A wholly owned subsidiary of Johnson &

Johnson employing some 2,200 employees and headquartered in Raritan, New Jersey, Ortho produced several pharmaceutical products, but Retin-A® was its most successful. In 1971 the FDA had approved Retin-A® as a topical treatment for acne, and granted Ortho approval to market, label, and promote the drug for that use only. Dr. Kligman told his medical counterpart at Ortho that the FDA would be a formidable opponent in gaining approval for the sale of Retin-A® as an antiaging cream. Kligman pointed out that "the NDA [new drug application] route would be lengthy, complicated, and likely to fail."[20] According to the recollection of Dr. George Thorne, Ortho's medical director of the dermatological division, Kligman's pessimism probably rested on his belief that, as an antiwrinkle cream, Retin-A® would be a cosmetic product and less acceptable to the FDA than a drug that mitigated disease.[21] Without the FDA's official clearance, a drug's financial success is dramatically lessened, if not doomed outright. Physicians could still prescribe "off-label" usage, but it was illegal for a company to promote off-label usage.

As an alternative to promotion, Kligman suggested the more studied, collegial, educational approach of using "his data base of some 300 to 400 patients" as "the basis of a monograph and/or a series of articles dealing with Retin-A® in the aging process."[22] In addition, he recommended that "a symposium [on] acne and other uses for the retinoids be planned" that would give a prominent part to the use of Retin-A® against aging skin. In brief, Kligman was suggesting a clever maneuver that would bypass FDA approval by orchestrating a propaganda campaign for the product targeted at consumers and dermatologists.

Kligman informed Ortho he was "quite willing to get behind this project" and volunteered to "help organize" the event at "the University of Pennsylvania or anywhere else." He was also prepared "to start on the project as soon as possible." The strategic meeting closed with both parties agreeing to explore Kligman's suggestions and to continue his "consultantship...for another year at the current stipend of $15,000."[23]

Ortho's corporate leadership adopted Kligman's advice: they would seek to increase Retin-A® sales by exploring new avenues of augmenting off-label sales of the drug. According to an October 1985 company document, they planned to spend "$1.6 million to implement a Retin-A® Educational Program" in an attempt to gain "acceptance by physicians and consumers of Retin-A®'s benefits for adult skin."[24] As the campaign notice explained: "to be most effective we need a program that makes our physicians receptive and drives consumers to dermatologists inquiring about Retin-A® benefits." Outreach programs would be designed to "recruit 1,000 dermatologists, across the U.S." to take part in special clinical trials on consumers and refer interested parties to a favorably disposed dermatologist in order to "close the consumer/dermatologist loop."

The extensive public relations campaign was a well-funded corporate initiative and adopted the motto: "A cover story on Retin-A® once a month, whether we need it or not!"[25] Numerous fashion and glamor magazines responded. In order to gain scholarly credibility, the PR campaign contracted with Boston University to sponsor a symposium in April 1986 on tretinoin's (Retin-A®'s) potential as an antiwrinkle medication. The day after the symposium, Boston University sponsored a follow-up seminar, "Cosmeceuticals: The Science and Beauty of Aging," featuring Dr. Albert M. Kligman delivering a lecture on Retin-A®'s use as a treatment for aging skin. Both the symposium and the seminar were financed by Ortho Pharmaceutical through its public relations firm, the Softness Group.

After the 1986 symposium, the Softness Group, at Ortho's direction, conducted an educational campaign that included a "consumer media tour" televising prominent dermatologists. The physicians were part of Ortho's stable of company-friendly medical show horses, each of whom received a $1,000 stipend to visit local television stations and "discuss the damaging effects of the sun, precancerous lesions, and the benefits of Retin-A®."[26] For example, the NBC television affiliate in Buffalo, New York, received a letter from the Softness Group in the fall of 1987, announcing the availability of Dr. Lynn Drake, a dermatologist, to discuss "tiny lines, melanin spots," and other harmful effects of the sun's rays.[27] Retin-A®, the most "effective" method yet discovered in combating "photodamage," was mentioned 8 times in the brief 7 paragraph letter.

As media tour participants, all of the dermatologists, including Drs. Kligman and Drake, received media training paid for by Ortho.

Each presentation was critiqued for Ortho executives by the Softness Group, who collected a library of transcripts and videotapes of physicians pitching the skin cream. Occasionally, they would offer suggestions for a physician's presentation. In one analysis designed to "improve Dr. Kligman's responses," the media advisers suggested "the focus [of his talks] should be on the product and not...collateral issues" such as off-label usage and financial rewards.[28] Ortho executives told Kligman to calm his enthusiastic rhetoric after hearing him comment on the *MacNeil/Lehrer News Hour* that Retin-A® sales had caused a "[literal] explosion, which has resulted in a very considerable sum of money that comes to our department in the form of royalties. We are swimming in cash."[29] A confidential internal company memo said pointedly that Kligman's comment "is one we could do without."[30]

The centerpiece of the public relations campaign, as the government would later frame it, was a lavish press conference at the Rainbow Room in Rockefeller Center, New York City. The January 1988 event was designed to "maximize the publicity" for a recently published paper in the *Journal of the American Medical Association.* The scholarly article by another Ortho-supported dermatologist, Dr. John Voorhees of the University of Michigan, discussed a study based on 30 patients that yielded the promising findings of topical tretinoin, the active ingredient in Retin-A®, in erasing fine wrinkles in the skin. News coverage was further enhanced by a "satellite media tour" that orchestrated interviews via satellite between Dr. Voorhees and television stations around the nation. For his services, Dr. Voorhees was paid $25,000 by Ortho Pharmaceutical.[31]

Ortho's Rainbow Room press conference and subsequent media blitz were extremely successful. Their key message points—that photodamage leads to premature wrinkling and skin cancer, and Retin-A® can reverse photodamage—were repeatedly broadcast across the country.[32] Not surprisingly, "Retin-A® sales skyrocketed." Prior to the Rainbow Room press conference, Retin-A® sales averaged $154,000 a day. After the media onslaught, sales approached $1.5 million a day.[33] Moreover, while 6 percent of Retin-A® sales had been attributed to off-label uses in 1987, in the following year, Ortho attributed 65 percent of Retin-A® sales to off-label uses.[34]

Although the media campaign was an "unprecedented" success resulting in windfall profits for Ortho and Kligman, it had attracted the eye of the FDA. Just two months after the Rainbow Room media blitz, the FDA "initiated an administrative proceeding to determine the scope and extent to which Ortho coordinated, controlled, and conducted the Retin-A® public relations campaign."[35] The FDA was not the only group intrigued by the well-organized, solidly-financed Retin-A® publicity campaign. Members of the media, particularly *60 Minutes* and *Money* magazine, began to investigate and publish stories exposing the Softness Group's connection to Ortho, the unlawful campaign to promote the unapproved use of Retin-A® as a treatment for photoaged skin, and the conflicts of interest of Drs. Gilchrist, Voorhees, and Kligman. In a thorough, eight-page article entitled "The Selling of Retin-A®," *Money* magazine pointed to the following items:

1. The pharmaceutical industry's increasing propensity to bypass clinical physicians and promote new prescription drugs directly to consumers through the popular press.

2. Major corporate publicity of medical researchers who abandon objectivity for corporate dollars in behalf of new products and lavish PR campaigns.

3. The extremely close relationships between pharmaceutical companies and doctors.

4. The shallow perusal by the general press of pharmaceutical company press releases in the quest for bold headlines.

5. The FDA's underfunded, understaffed administrative situation in the face of well-organized corporate initiatives and sophisticated publicity techniques.[36]

The end result of the revealing article was a collective black-eye for the pharmaceutical industry, dermatologists, the American Medical Association, and its esteemed journal.

II

The negative electronic and print coverage that Ortho started to receive in 1989—the year in which Ortho filed a new drug application with the FDA for Renova® (the antiwrinkle variation of Retin-A®)—was not the only troublesome problem for the company. Congressional hearings had begun, as well as a nasty civil suit that involved Dr. Kligman, Johnson & Johnson, and the University of Pennsylvania.

Congressman Ted Weiss of New York initiated hearings on off-label usage in the pharmaceutical industry, with Retin-A® playing a prominent role. According to Diana Zuckerman of the committee's investigative staff, they were able to "put together" a case concerning Ortho's Retin-A® campaign.[37] "We got videotapes and documents quoting Kligman on campaign strategy [aimed at promoting] this off-label usage," says Zuckerman. The committee believed they had enough evidence to implicate Ortho in a promotional campaign. Furthermore, the committee questioned Retin-A®'s effectiveness. "We said Retin-A® was highly questionable. The committee wanted to know how objective were the measures in judging the drug." They understood that its use was "leading to puffiness and pink skin, but was the skin younger, or more elastic and the wrinkles hidden?" A number of critics were beginning to wonder if Retin-A® did not so much remove wrinkles as hide them under irritated skin that was puffed up and smoother.

The more emotionally charged problem for Dr. Kligman was the legal confrontation with his longtime employer, the University of Pennsylvania, which began on May 10, 1989, when University Patents, Inc., a Connecticut firm that administered patents for the university, sued Kligman and Johnson & Johnson. The suit claimed Kligman "breached its patent policy."[38] At stake were the millions of dollars that were expected to be earned on the highly publicized antiwrinkle cream, Renova®, that was awaiting FDA approval.

The university and the patent company claimed that Kligman had violated the school's conflict of interest and intellectual property rules when he had applied for a patent in his own name for Renova® and quietly gave a commercial license to Johnson & Johnson. The university had no doubt that the new drug, Renova®, along with its predecessor Retin-A®, had been developed on the university's campus, in its own laboratories, and with its own scientific equipment. The university's attorneys argued that Kligman colluded with Johnson & Johnson to deprive the university of its rightful share of profits in the following ways:

1. Kligman breached the Patent Policy on August 28, 1981, when he filed for a patent for the photoaging invention in his own name.

2. Kligman had consulting agreements with Johnson & Johnson in the early to mid-1970s that demonstrate further concealment and indifference to the university's conflict of interest policy.

3. Kligman violated the "1967 tri-party agreement by entering into a separate agreement (one of the consulting agreements) that provided him with a royalty on Retin-A® sales."[39]

The university's attorneys presented examples of Dr. Kligman's deception in his dealings with university officials. The attorneys relied on letters written in October 1985 and February 1986 to Dr. Gerald Lazarus, chairman of the dermatology department, describing "campaigns to increase the sales of Retin-A®" and "a legal campaign to obtain an extension of the patent on Retin-A®."[40] Kligman said success in this venture would result in a "bonanza for our department" and potential "royalties for another 10 years." (He added to Lazarus, "I also want you to know that I am bearing the legal costs myself. I may turn out to be an angel yet!")

The university attorneys claimed that "at the time he wrote this letter, Dr. Kligman was not engaged in a campaign to extend the prior Retin-A® patent. Rather, he had filed an application for a new product and had received notice that it would be approved after a successful effort to convince the relevant authorities that his current discovery was sufficiently different from the original one."[41]

Throughout the 1980s, Kligman had shepherded his new chemical composition through a legal minefield—from filing for a new patent, to an arrangement with Johnson & Johnson to sell them exclusive patent rights, to obtaining the new patent in 1986—so that when the original Retin-A® patent expired, he would have the newer, more lucrative one. Patent No. 4,603,146 issued in July 1986, allowed him to be "sole owner" and gave him the freedom to license the invention. He quickly licensed it with Johnson & Johnson and gave them exclusive rights to make, use, and sell the new product. In return, he received the favorable royalty rate of a sliding scale of 5 percent, 3 percent and 1 percent on U.S. sales. "The university was not made a party to the agreement."[42]

Meanwhile, Ortho's antiwrinkle cream campaign was in full swing and FDA investigators were busy building a case against Ortho on off-label marketing. At the same time, the news media were describing "[a] new wrinkle in [the] Retin-A® case," and observing that "the purpose of academic research no longer is to advance knowledge, but to advance profits."[43]

III

The court battle over Retin-A® patent rights and its attendant press coverage could not have come at a worse time. In December 1990 the civil suit brought to light an interoffice memo written in 1983 by Dr. George Thorne, the medical director for Ortho's dermatology division. FDA investigators found the 7-year-old memo particularly interesting because it disclosed the meeting between Thorne and Kligman in which Kligman had proposed that Ortho sponsor an academic symposium to "launch" Retin-A® as an antiwrinkle treatment, prior to FDA approval. For FDA officials, congressmen, and investigative journalists, the memo represented a smoking gun, a critical piece of evidence that revealed the intent and scope of the Retin-A® off-label marketing campaign. The FDA requested a grand jury investigation, and a congressional staff member told a reporter for the university's daily newspaper that the memo indicated that "Ortho Pharmaceuticals circumvented FDA regulations."[44] The CBS program *60 Minutes* rebroadcast their earlier Retin-A® story, and this time they discussed the damaging memo. In a succinct corporate reply, Ortho called the memo a "speculative conversation between two physicians about potential activities involving Retin-A® .025% cream that subsequently never occurred....This memo does not reflect the marketing plans of Ortho Pharmaceutical Corporation."[45]

During the last days of 1990, a New Jersey grand jury investigation was launched by the U.S. Department of Justice. It was designed to determine "whether Ortho, its employees and agents hired by Ortho, engaged in a conspiracy to defraud the FDA and the public by unlawfully promoting Retin-A® for unapproved purposes."[46]

IV

Because of the evidence contained in the 1983 memo, federal investigators worked hard to get more information from Ortho. FDA agents made unannounced evening visits to the homes of two company executives, Dr. George Thorne and Lester W. Riley, the head of Ortho's dermatology division. The investigators gained little information, but when they left, "high ranking Ortho representatives were told of the visits and the reason for the visits."[47] By early the next morning, January 3, 1991, word of the FDA visits to the homes of Ortho's employees had spread throughout the company's administrative offices, and employees were working feverishly to destroy all documents related to the Retin-A® public relations programs. Throughout the day and evening, employees were recruited to assist in the shredding. When employees expressed reluctance, they were reminded of Ortho's document retention policy, but it was a sham— only the Retin-A® items from previous years were destroyed. Within Ortho's Public Affairs Group, a similar effort was underway. Employees were told to clean out their files and take home videotapes showing the company-funded consumer media tour. By the end of the day on January 3, thousands of documents had been shredded and numerous videotapes had been destroyed or hidden in the homes of company employees. The U.S. attorney general would later argue, "There is no doubt that the expedited destruction of documents was non-routine and that it was done to ensure that the FDA and other government investigators would not obtain those documents."[48]

On that same day, an assistant U.S. attorney informed a Johnson & Johnson attorney that the government had opened a criminal investigation into the promotion of Retin-A®. By 4:43 P.M. a grand jury subpoena had been faxed to the corporation's general counsel. The subpoena ordered Johnson & Johnson (including its subsidiary Ortho) to produce a lengthy list of items, most of which had just been destroyed. The records that remained were generally innocuous and of little importance; the critical documents that had demonstrated how Ortho orchestrated and directed the public relations firms in the Retin-A® media campaign were gone.

V

Meanwhile, the civil suit, *University Patents, Inc. v. Albert M. Kligman and Johnson & Johnson*, had gone through several motions to dismiss, lengthy discovery sessions, and charges against Kligman's attorney for breach of professional ethics. The trial had divided the University of Pennsylvania community as various college officials and faculty members became pitted against one another over what Albert Kligman had told them about his wonder cream, and when he "discovered [it]...while treating inmates at...Holmesburg Prison in the 1960s."[49]

Suddenly, in early March 1992, the legal battle over the patent culminated in an out-of-court settlement that apparently left the parties reasonably content. The specific terms of the agreement were not disclosed, but Ortho spokespersons proudly announced: "Johnson & Johnson [has retained] exclusive ownership of the patent rights to Retin-A®, but will pay royalties to University Patents, Inc. and to Penn."[50] The royalties, it was assumed, would be based on future Renova® sales. Past royalties on Retin-A® sales were lost forever.

Kligman was pleased the legal fight was finally over and expressed benevolence for his employer. He was reported as saying: "I didn't know Retin-A® was going to yield all this wealth. I'm delighted, because it's my way of paying back this university that trained me, educated me, gave me a chance to grow, and didn't hold me back."[51]

VI

At approximately the same time that the civil suit was being settled, the FDA was examining the scientific claims of Retin-A® as a wrinkle remover. Before and after photographs of subjects treated with the alleged antiwrinkle cream were unimpressive although they appeared to show better results than other facial creams on the market. Many physicians questioned the authenticity of the photos. The FDA's Alan Lisook recalls that "the photographs were not the best."[52] The photos showing the dramatic improvement from the use of Retin-A® "seemed to be taken in a different way." Kligman himself expressed amazement at Dr. Voorhees's initial sets of photographs. "I can't get

the kinds of results that Voorhees is reporting," Kligman told newspaper writers.[53] "Maybe it's creative photography—what the hell. I
don't know what he's doing, but it just doesn't seem right to me." Still,
the FDA advisory committee leaned toward approving a new-use designation for Retin-A®, and Ortho had visions of advertising "a fountain of youth in a tube" under the name Renova®, but the FDA scientists were more skeptical of the claimed benefits. Furthermore, the
FDA had decided to withhold its decision until the grand jury and
justice department had concluded their own criminal investigation.

In December 1992, Johnson & Johnson attorneys made the surprise
announcement that company officials had taken part in shredding
documents pertinent to the case. For the next two years, the federal
grand jury conducted detailed inquiries and collected voluminous
data in anticipation of charging Ortho and its officials with obstruction of justice. Finally, in January 1995, aware that Retin-A®'s new
antiwrinkle status was held captive to interminable legal proceedings,
corporate officials announced that they would plead guilty.

On January 11, 1995, District Judge William G. Bassler asked Jed
Rakoff, attorney for Ortho Pharmaceutical, a series of questions:

1. In or about early January 1991, was a federal grand jury conducting an
   investigation into whether Ortho had unlawfully promoted Retin-A® for
   photoaging and for other unapproved indications?

2. On or about January 3rd, 1991, did Ortho...knowingly and corruptly persuade, and attempt to persuade the employees...to destroy, mutilate, and
   conceal documents and other objects in the possession, custody, and control
   of Ortho and the Public Affairs Group?

3. Did representatives of Ortho knowingly and corruptly persuade the
   employees...with intent to cause and induce them to destroy, mutilate, and
   conceal documents and other objects with the intent to impair the integrity
   and availability of those documents and objects for use in an official proceeding?[54]

Ortho's legal representative replied "Yes" to each of the questions.

On April 10, 1995, Judge Bassler ruled that for "[putting] itself
above the law...Ortho, a company whose business activities can have
an impact on the public health," would be fined a maximum
$500,000 for each of the ten felonies charged for a total of $5 million

plus $2.5 million in restitution.[55] Although the $7.5 million fine was one of the largest ever paid for an FDA violation, it was modest in comparison to the millions of dollars Ortho had illegally gained while promoting Retin-A®'s off-label usage. Judge Bassler was well aware of this discrepancy: "There is no doubt that Ortho will be able to pay promptly such a fine and restitution without imposing any undue burden on the company." He added, however, "I am hopeful that the sentence will send the correct message to the entire corporate community, particularly firms in the medical field....The maximum $500,000 per count sentence alone may not be enough to deter a corporation bent on obstructing justice from engaging in a criminal obstruction, but it at least puts such a corporation on notice that they can expect a maximum sentence to be imposed where warranted."[56]

For Kenneth Jost, assistant director of the Office of Consumer Litigation for the U.S. Justice Department and prosecution cocounsel, Ortho's admission of guilt in the obstruction of justice allegation was a considerable victory. "The fine was one of the most significant for a Food and Drug case," says Jost.[57] But ultimately, the financial penalty for obstruction of justice enabled Ortho to escape the original accusation that it had illegally promoted an off-label use for a specific medication. The illegal promotion charge never culminated in another high profile trial. Jost says, "We investigated the whole marketing of Retin-A®...and the tension between education and promotion. There's a fine line there. We decided against prosecution."

The government did prosecute, however, the person they believed orchestrated the document destruction campaign: Lester W. Riley, Jr., the manager and the highest-ranking employee of the dermatological division of Ortho Pharmaceutical. According to the grand jury indictment, Riley "knowingly, willfully, and unlawfully [conspired]...to defraud an agency of the United States and...authorized" Ortho employees "to destroy documents and objects relating to the Retin-A® public relations campaign."[58]

Since Ortho had already admitted to shredding the documents, Riley's conviction for ordering the destruction seemed likely. But Riley's defense was fundamentally simple: he claimed he had given an innocuous order that had been misinterpreted by an overzealous aide. Riley's critical comment, "Now would be a good time to clean out the files," and the testimony of two Riley subordinates who allegedly followed his orders and destroyed the files, became the centerpiece of the trial.[59] Riley was acquitted of the charges. Ken Jost remembers, "We knew it was a difficult trial," but they felt obligated to pursue it. "The not guilty verdict was not a surprise. One woman's memory had deteriorated before the trial," and the critical statement "take care of the files" was interpreted differently by various people.

Within a month of the 1995 decision in the Riley case, the FDA announced that Renova® had been approved for sale. But this verdict was not a total victory for Ortho. The company had hoped to advertise Renova® as a skin cure-all with medicinal properties capable of repairing a host of both severe and minor problems, but the FDA allowed Ortho to claim only that Renova® can be "used in the mitigation of fine wrinkles, mottled hyper-pigmentation, and tactile roughness of facial skin in patients." Furthermore, these accomplishments have "not been established in people greater than 50 years of age" or those "with moderately to heavily pigmented skin"; any improvement lasts only as long as the retinoid cream is used; and Renova®'s safety has not been proved beyond 48 weeks. The FDA insisted that every tube, costing approximately $75, carry a disclaimer: "Renova® does not eliminate wrinkles, repair sun damaged skin, reverse photoaging, or restore a more youthful or younger dermal histologic pattern." Despite such restrictions, prominent ads describing Renova® as "the only prescription medication proven to treat fine wrinkles caused by sunlight and time" and the only one "proven to give skin a smoother texture and rosier glow" pervade the beauty and health sections of many magazines.

There remains a broad range of medical opinion about the drug's wrinkle, reduction capabilities. Many dermatologists swear by it, and one, Dr. Faria Mescar, refers to it as "magic."[60] Others express reservations. Dr. Gerald Wachs says, "Retin-A® is standard therapy for acne. I use it 15 times per day for patients...but I'm less inclined to deal with it for other things....wrinkles are cosmetics."[61] Dr. Frederich Urbach says he has "used very little of Retin-A®" because the drug's powerful irritation led him to seek other substitutes for his patients.[62] "When you start using it, the skin inflames and becomes tender and raw, and some of my patients did not like it. It was too rough. I found other drugs that work as well and did not have the initial harsh impact."

The success of Retin-A® and Renova® is a testament not only to our fascination with perpetual youth, but also to the career of one physician-researcher. Albert Kligman's driving curiosity, consistent knack for cutting bureaucratic and ethical corners, and daring ability to subject patients to conditions more prudent investigators rejected, have been rewarded many times over. Others, of course, benefited as well, especially the University of Pennsylvania which allowed its creative but prodigal dermatologist the freedom to explore scientific and ethical boundaries.

Nine

"A Conspiracy of Silence."

Maimonides, the 12th-century philosopher and physician, advised his colleagues to treat patients not merely as the means to the acquisition of knowledge, but as valuable in themselves. Eight hundred years later, another physician, Dr. Albert M. Kligman, advised his colleagues and taught his students that "rules don't apply to geniuses."[1] For Kligman, the benchmark of a successful career in medicine is medical knowledge and the wealth it can generate.

This utilitarian approach to research subjects, combined with equal doses of personal drive, intellectual brilliance, and entrepreneurial skill, allowed Dr. Kligman to establish a formidable record of accomplishment and financial success. Unfortunately, a large portion of that celebrated and lucrative medical research career was wrung, literally, from the sweat of prison inmates anxious to earn money to provide for themselves. An uninformed and desperate group of prisoners met an unrestrained and ambitious doctor, and Holmesburg Prison became one of postwar America's largest, nontherapeutic, human research factories. Many American prisons housed medical research labs during the Cold War. Few, if any, involved as many test subjects in as wide a variety of experimental protocols for as many years as Holmesburg did. Even more remarkable is how such a large and intricate operation in a public facility went so long unnoticed and unchallenged. Several reasons for this lapse in social and political sensitivity suggest themselves, beginning with this nation's failure to take seriously the Nuremberg Code.

I

Intended by its earliest settlers to be "a city on a hill," a moral north star to an amoral world, America has long been among the most insular and self-satisfied of nations. So although three American judges at the Nazi Doctors Trial promoted the principles of the Nuremberg Code and sentenced Nazi physicians to death in its name, it may be no surprise that the Nuremberg Code "was buried soon after its birth" in America.[2] In the opinion of the American medical comunity, this new code of medical ethics was designed for Nazi physicians: "written for the specific purpose of preventing brutal excesses from being committed or excused in the name of science." As the assistant dean of Harvard Medical School told an administrative board when applying for a military research grant in 1961, the Nuremberg Code "is not necessarily pertinent to or adequate for the conduct of medical research in the United States."[3]

In fact, the view that American medicine deserved an exception to the Code was expressed during the Nuremberg trial before the Code itself was drafted. Dr. Andrew C. Ivy, "the conscience of U.S. science,"[4] and the prosecution's key witness on medical ethics, argued on the witness stand that prison research in America was "ideal" and "all subjects have been volunteers in the absence of coercion in any form." These pronouncements were endorsed a short while later by the American Medical Association and prominently printed in its respected journal for all physicians to digest.[5]

The physicians interviewed for this book began their medical careers immediately after the war. They report that medical ethics were not taught in medical school, much less emphasized, and the Nuremberg Code was never mentioned. Nazi medicine was a horrible but distant medical aberration that could never happen here. Indeed, the moral superiority of American research was the received norm by which Nazi doctors were judged. In addition, the reasoning continued, because scientific progress was best achieved through independence and autonomy, and since Nazi science had flourished under governmental intrusion and control, American doctors deserved deference and encouragement, not oversight and outside management.[6] Perhaps to head off these possible controlling influences, the

American Medical Association adopted its own "Rules of Human Experimentation" (written by the ubiquitous Dr. Andrew Ivy) prescribing that:

1. the voluntary consent of the person on whom the experiment is to be performed [must be obtained].

2. the danger of each experiment must be previously investigated by animal experimentation.

3. the experiment must be performed under proper medical protection and management.[7]

At the same time, prestigious medical journals published articles reporting and recommending the use of vulnerable, institutionalized children or prisoners as "ideal" test subjects. For physician-researchers, there appeared to be few constraints. Not remarkably, then, the next two decades saw numerous scientific advances, but at the expense of the Nuremberg Code, the AMA's own code, and the health and dignity of thousands of human subjects. When Dr. Henry Beecher published his attack on unethical research practices he met a firestorm of ridicule, as if he were a wild-eyed radical seeking to revolutionize the medical profession's procedures, scuttle tradition, and turn decision-making over to codes of conduct written by government bureaucrats. The Harvard-based anesthesiologist had pointed out that a "more reliable safeguard" against unethical research methods was the "presence of an intelligent, informed, conscientious, compassionate, responsible investigator."[8] But medical precedents, an insular AMA, and a growing profit motive fueled by lucrative research contracts made any reform impossible.

Accordingly, the Holmesburg medical research program originated and thrived well after the creation by American jurists of the Nuremberg Code. The principles of the Code, particularly the first principle covering "voluntary consent," which stressed "free power of choice" and the absence of "any element of force...or constraint or coercion" should have prevented American scientific investigators from pursuing medical initiatives on imprisoned populations. In fact, the opposite occurred. The U.S. medical establishment, guided by a research ethic that rewarded scientific triumphs over the concepts of patients' rights and subjects' autonomy, chose to enrich itself from corporate and government research largess. And human experiments, which brought this largess to life, flourished. The doctors who entered Holmesburg Prison a few short years after Nuremberg were conditioned to see the mass of idle humanity before them as a "fertile field" of investigatory opportunity. As Albert M. Kligman graphically framed it, prisoners had become a new experimental resource, they had become "acres of skin."

II

As we have seen, throughout the postwar years, there developed a disturbing willingness to experiment on society's most vulnerable members: the mentally retarded, the mentally ill, hospital patients, and prisoners. Liberties were taken, ethical corners cut, and sensitivity relinquished not by the collective medical community, but by ambitious and occasionally amoral individual physicians and researchers. One of these was Dr. Albert M. Kligman.

The healing/harming paradox that enveloped Kligman and his medical research program left its mark—literally and professionally—on all its participants. As Kligman's research program—which was established to investigate diseases and to train residents in dermatology at the University of Pennsylvania—grew, it strayed from its mission. In time, no protocol was too risky, no relationship too troubling, no code immune to violating. By the mid-1960s, Kligman had developed a national reputation for performing human studies and had cultivated an impressive list of corporate clients. A new medical culture emerged in which the researchers' ambitions had clearly become as important as the prisoners' well-being.

The effect that such a large and profitable human research operation had on Kligman's students is incalculable. According to Dr. Paul Gross, a former colleague: "No students questioned his tactics or methods. They were all in awe of him."[9] Students were mesmerized by their professor's theatrical lecture hall presentations, intellectual brilliance, and personal flair. Dr. A. Bernard Ackerman remembers that Kligman claimed he was quoting the French physician, scholar, and researcher Claude Bernard when he frequently boasted, "The only reason I do the experiments is to please the critics. I know the answers ahead of time."[10] (Ackerman thinks it unlikely that Claude Bernard ever said it, but very likely that the sentiment appealed to Kligman.) And Kligman's unique prison studies only further illuminated his star qualities. He became the role model for an entire generation of dermatologists hoping to emulate their mentor's exciting and stylish approach to life and medicine. An avid tennis player, motorcycle and airplane enthusiast, and self-proclaimed womanizer, Kligman could also generate ideas that inspired his students. He had something special; some called it "pizzazz." Dr. Ackerman says, "Kligman was the most interesting man in dermatology. Nobody was as dashing and as exciting. He was the dominant figure—he was intriguing and was alive intellectually. All of the residents modeled themselves after Kligman." Students were captivated and many planned their professional careers with Kligman's maxims and achievements in mind. Former students, Dr. William Epstein and Dr. Howard Maibach directed research clinics at San Quentin and Vacaville State Prisons and were happily ensconced at those sites until the 1970s, when their research projects fell victim to changing attitudes and the bad publicity fostered by Jessica Mitford's exposé.[11]

Kligman's influence combined with his willingness to spend vast amounts of time, energy, and resources on wrinkle-reduction remedies and other cosmetic initiatives changed the study of dermatology. For Dr. Kligman and many of his students, fostering the cosmetics industry was the same as practicing real medicine. Money and fame had come to replace more worthwhile endeavors for "Kligman's boys." Thus, a generation of dermatological investigators were driven to become highly paid laboratory heroes. The impact of this phenomenon even extended beyond U.S. borders. "He's one of the best known dermatologists in Europe," says Dr. C. Stuttgen, a long-time German observer who also noted that Kligman was "not a person filled with discipline," but enjoyed "[playing] the artist in dermatology."[12] For the master's closest disciples—and those who perfected their craft at Holmesburg—the pursuit of career advancement, publications, lucrative contracts, and fame, became the goals of their professional careers.

As far as the medical profession as a whole was concerned, Kligman's work and the Holmesburg research program were acceptable. In fact, many in the medical community found the clinical testing program at the prison exceedingly attractive. Enormous sums of money changed hands, but under Dr. Kligman's bold direction, captives of the county's criminal justice system were not only sentenced to serve time in prison, but subjected to misguided science as well. Kligman's blatant medical abuses allow the Holmesburg experiments to be compared to the barbarity and sadism of Auschwitz and Dachau. His defenders, among them Dr. Frederich Urbach, denounce Nazi analogies as extreme, arguing that "Albert is not a scoundrel," just an "enthusiast" who "gets carried away by his enthusiasm....You have to consider the social aspects of the time. There was no such thing as medical ethics. No one taught it."[13] Maybe, but it now seems understandable enough that for someone who took the Hippocratic oath, Kligman's professional behavior was itself problematic. In his zeal to earn money and fame, and in his impatience with procedure, Kligman violated the Hippocratic injunction to do no harm to the test subjects under his care.

III

For the University of Pennsylvania School of Medicine, the first medical school to be established in the New World, and where Dr. Kligman spent his entire career, the Gilded Age of Research Medicine paid off handsomely. The university fostered Albert Kligman and an "incredibly strong line-up of stars" during the 1950s and 1960s.[14] Clarence Livingood, Howard Maibach, Bernard Ackerman, Herbert Mescon, Martin Carter, and John Strauss all passed through the university's dermatological program. The university allowed the members of its medical community to go unsupervised and enjoy the freedom to determine individual research goals and methods because those who chose to work for well-heeled clients helped support the school. While some colleagues who worried about Kligman's relationships and subsequent experiments learned to look the other way and not ask embarrassing questions, not all of them even worried. Dr. Walter Shelley, chair of the dermatology department, recalled that he "was fully aware of Kligman's outside work and never considered it improper."[15] Research ethics, which should have been a core element of their program, were de-emphasized, the better to "reap the benefits" of Holmesburg's burgeoning human experimentation program. Even as the years passed and troubling aspects of that research program began to receive media attention, the university was not prepared to jettison Dr. Kligman and his ethically bankrupt but economically enriching prison research. As Dr. Shelley observes: "Kligman brought in all this money. Millions and millions of dollars....In the beginning,...the university considered work with pharmaceutical companies unsuitable....But the pendulum was starting to swing [and] Kligman was on the cutting edge."[16]

In addition to the corrupting influence of money was a more troubling and deeper dilemma: the money poured in not from farsighted investments or wealthy alumni, but through the use of vulnerable institutionalized populations as test subjects in medical experiments. By proclaiming that "the employment of human test subjects is ideal" in reference to retarded children, and declaring, "We have not been alive enough to the wealth of test material that there is in penitentiaries," respected University of Pennsylvania Medical School professors were fostering a research atmosphere that rejected both the Hippocratic Oath and the Nuremberg Code.[17] Cheap and available test subjects locked behind bars and in other human warehouses answered the investigators' chief concerns: how to collect a large enough sample population to give validity to an experiment's results, and how to maintain control of that sample. The exploitation of vulnerable Americans had become the bedrock of the university's famous and widely respected dermatology department. Albert Kligman may have been the catalyst for, and the most accomplished at, this shameful practice, but he was by no means alone.

IV

Unfortunately, the field of corrections, as it is euphemistically called, has never attracted the best and brightest in society. Many prison wardens and superintendents during the period of this study began their careers as guards, and even the better educated and more sophisticated officials were susceptible to a naive overreliance on medical experts. Too often, wardens had little more information about the experiments the prisoners were about to embark on than the inmates themselves, but they had already delegated their responsibility as supervisors for their wards to the impressive, well-spoken men in white lab coats. In their deference to the medical profession and lack of appropriate concern for the prisoners housed on their cell blocks, prison wardens collaborated with the medical profession in the creation of numerous human rights abuses. The sheer size of the program—that at times saw 90 percent of the prison population participating in one experiment or another—staggered inmates, guards, and doctors alike. "There must have been a payoff to the warden to allow all the testing," speculates Dr. Gross.[18]

In Philadelphia, the history of prisoner experimentation is fairly typical. Superintendents (Baldi and Hendrick initially, and much later, Aytch) allowed physicians to establish medical research programs with the understanding that the prisoners would be paid, the experiments would be relatively harmless, and medical science a potential beneficiary. Though all three superintendents are deceased, their subordinates find it difficult to believe that their superiors were aware of the nuances of the testing program and the inherent dangers involved. This may be, but the testing "certainly disrupted the prison routine,"[19] and the incidence of burned, rash-covered, and disoriented inmate-volunteers were too numerous to go unnoticed. Observation could, and should, have prompted prison officials to ask the doctors pointed questions and to become familiar with the nuances. Many staff members had questions about the experiments that were a daily presence throughout the city's three-prison system, but in a rigid, paramilitary organization, employees were trained to take orders, respect authority, and not make waves. There is no record of any staff member—either uniformed or civilian—ever raising concerns or protesting the nature of the research underway during the program's many years of operation. The exploitation of prisoners was as widely accepted as it was recognized.

In search of data on the effect of drugs on humans, Philadelphia's county prison system supplied the key ingredient sophisticated laboratories in both the private and public sectors lacked: human guinea pigs. R. J. Reynolds in North Carolina, Dow Chemical in Michigan, the U.S. Army in Maryland, the CIA in Virginia, Johnson & Johnson in New Jersey, and numerous pharmaceutical companies around the country, all came to Philadelphia to see Dr. Kligman because at Holmesburg bodies were readily available. Their interests varied greatly, from smoking's impact on the body's triptophan to dioxin's effects on skin, from incapacitating mind-altering drugs for the Army to mind-control drugs for the CIA; but they all believed their research goals could be met by gaining access to a county jail in Philadelphia. The relationships that formed over the years made reputations and lined the pockets of everyone involved. Everyone, of course, but the prisoners who traded blistered backs, a week's nausea, or much worse for "chump change," a tiny fraction of the profits paid to Kligman and the University of Pennsylvania.

V

Of course, there is little doubt that the Holmesburg human guinea pigs acquiesced in their own exploitation. Uneducated and isolated, desperately short of money, the inmates of Holmesburg Prison were an easy target for medical mercenaries looking for test subjects. A drowning person does not ask penetrating questions about a life raft. So too did most Holmesburg test subjects keep their questions about the tests to themselves. Some may have decided to believe that the "perfume tests" were harmless, but many understood they were gambling with their health and safety without knowing the risks and without giving genuine, uncoerced, informed consent. The university researchers at Holmesburg understood the setup. Dr. Gerd Plewig, a former resident, recalls the concept of informed consent as a recent development. "During these days uninformed patients was the rule. We told them about the tests, but nothing like we do today."[20] He says that there were few restraints on physicians or their research, and the gradual development of experimental restrictions came years later.

Not surprisingly, few, if any, prisoners volunteered to advance science, display patriotism, or demonstrate altruism. The better educated and the better-off financially an inmate was, the less likely he was to make himself available for the experiments. Upon their release from prison, the former test volunteers rarely participated in free-world clinical studies. The freedom to earn money in other ways—both legal and illegal—lessened their enthusiasm for becoming human guinea pigs again; whenever, or as soon as, the men of

Holmesburg were able finally to give the informed consent all medical guidelines mandate, they withheld it.

Today, the physical and psychological scars from their days as
Holmesburg volunteers are ever present. Embarrassed by the linger-
ing marks on their bodies and pained by their memories, they regret
past decisions and have only disdain for the eminent men of medicine who offered them "money for a piece of their skin." Johnnie
Williams is typical of many former African-American prisoners who
feel used and claim they will never be able to trust doctors again.
Many former test subjects and their families now regard the medical
profession as torturers rather than healers.

As we approach the 21st century, the nation's prison population
continues to grow. The needs of today's prisoners differ little from
those of a generation ago. Despite the passing years and much that
we have learned about the scientific abuse of vulnerable populations, many of the conditions that persuaded prisoners to choose
dehumanizing medical experiments as a source of income continue
to exist. Nearly a quarter century after the Holmesburg experiments
ended, the 6,000 prisoners in the Philadelphia prison system still
have no way to provide for themselves and would probably "volunteer" once again if Albert M. Kligman's program were available.
Prisoners will only be able to exercise their inalienable rights of
truly informed consent when opportunites for prison employment
expand and increase.

VI

The Holmesburg experiments took place before the rise of investigative
journalism, and the media, the government, and the public in general,
neither knew nor cared about the events occurring daily within the
walls of the old city jail. On those rare occasions when the local and
national press did print articles regarding the experiments on humans,
they remained superficial and laudatory. Beginning in the mid-1950s
with *Life* magazine's account of Kligman's poison ivy experiments,
local newspaper stories depicted Kligman as a hero on the front lines
of science and medicine. The test subjects were described as his willing allies in such articles as "Prisoners Volunteer To Save Lives," and
"Prisoners Aid Research, 75% Here Act as Medical Guinea Pigs."[21]

Journalists and assignment desk editors acted unaware of and untroubled by the potential for abuse inherent in such an environment. Even when the Philadelphia district attorney's investigation revealed that sodomy was the price paid by weaker inmates to those stronger for the opportunity to be included in Kligman's research program, reporters never revisited the endemic corruption caused by the power of the research program. Kligman and his medical research operation were affecting the lives of thousands of Philadelphians, but no newsroom in the city sent a reporter to Holmesburg while the experiments continued until well into the next decade.

Governmental officials too, were either unaware of or uninterested in a prison research program well known in medical and pharmaceutical circles, particularly one in which all parties seemed to benefit. The partnership between the prison system and the University of Pennsylvania had been sealed with a handshake. Not until 1969, 15 years after Kligman established his lab, did the city controller of Philadelphia recommend a formal, signed contract. The prisoners could have told any government official enough about the research program to have it abolished. But for 20 years, through experiment after experiment, no one bothered to examine the effects on the prisoners of the research program. The FDA bowed to pressure from a former surgeon general and a professor emeritus at the University of Pennsylvania medical school who stepped in to oversee Kligman's sloppy, dangerous, and unscientific methods; but Kligman was reinstated as an approved FDA researcher and the profitable program continued. The Army found inadequate facilities and contaminated experiment sites; Kligman was required to revise his procedures and establish new sites in trailers before the Army granted a contract for its experiments. The EPA looked the other way and the AEC was duped. No government agency—knowing the inherent dangers to the prisoners in sloppy methods when drugs with unknowable effects are being tested—questioned that the prisoners could be exercising informed, uncoerced consent. Only Dow Chemical irrevocably canceled a contract because of the risks that Kligman took in his human trials. In the end it was lawsuits from individual prisoners that highlighted abuses that could no longer be ignored. As officials and reporters watched from a distance, prisoners themselves brought an end to medical research at Holmesburg by putting their hands in the wallets of the university and the city.

VII

In 1946, the leaders of the American Medical Association responded to information about the full range of brutalities committed by Nazi physicians during World War II by raising a "standard of conduct compatible with the nature of the profession."[22] An editorial in the *Journal of the American Medical Association* underscored the "Principles of Medical Ethics" and the qualities required for the "art of healing." A physician, they cautioned their membership, "must keep himself pure in character and conform to a high standard of morals."

That 1946 call for ethical vigiliance on the part of the profession was followed by three decades of physicians abusing the rights of patients on a scale unparalleled in American medical history, unaccompanied by protests or sanctions by the AMA. "It couldn't happen in America" we reassured ourselves about medical practices in Nazi Germany. But intolerable medical practices were practiced on vulnerable populations in America, without the support of the political culture or the despotic leadership that captivated Germany under the Third Reich, without any protest from the AMA, which prides itself on its ability to regulate itself.

History suggests that we are as susceptible to abusing our socially and economically disenfranchised citizens as any other nation. If, as many believe, a democracy is only as strong as the respect accorded its weakest members, we must work to assure that neither these abuses nor the "conspiracy of silence"[23] that makes them possible ever happen again. We must do this not only for the benefit of the powerless, but also for the benefit of society as a whole. As philosopher Hans Jonas cautioned during the height of the human experimentation debate:

> Let us not forget that progress is an optional goal, not an unconditional commitment, and that its tempo in particular, compulsive as it may become, has nothing sacred about it. Let us also remember that a slower progress in the conquest of disease would not threaten society...but that society would indeed be threatened by the erosion of those moral values whose loss, possibly caused by too ruthless a pursuit of scientific progress, would make its most dazzling triumphs not worth having.[24]

Acknowledgments

The decision to jettison my job in the Philadelphia Sheriff's Office in order to research and write the history of the Holmesburg Prison medical experiments had more to do with faith and commitment than prudent decision-making. Without a regular income (except for some part-time teaching at Temple University) or a book contract, and with the gradual diminution of my savings, the project took on the appearance of a less than rewarding personal crusade. Fortunately, my mother proved to be an anchor of stability and a source of support. I will always be indebted to her for the unflinching faith she had in me, even though I gave her cause to doubt my historical quest on numerous occasions.

There are several individuals who deserve to be singled out for their assistance in this project. I thank my editor, Heidi Freund, for her quick recognition of the importance of the book's subject matter, and for the steadfast support and guidance she provided throughout the publication process. Appreciation is also extended to Ilene Kalish and Lai Moy for their commitment to this project. I would like to thank Amy Stackhouse, Sarita Sahni, Ron Longe, Debora Hilu, and John McHale.

I also owe a special debt of gratitude to A. Bernard Ackerman, whose medical reputation is exceeded only by his desire for the moral exercise of medicine. Dr. Ackerman proved a valuable ally, a witness to the experiments, a stalwart supporter of this historical investigation, a morale booster, and a manscript editor of the work in progress.

I am grateful to those scholars, writers, lawyers, and archivists who generously shared their research, knowledge, and thoughts with me: Susan Lederer, Robert Proctor, Arthur Caplan, Jonathan

Moreno, Evelyn Shuster, Jay Katz, Ann Diestel, Kenneth Jost, Tom Maeder, Suzanne White Junod, David Oshinsky, James Ketchum, Larry Cohan, Cathy Bucher, and Dick Florschutz.

I am also indebted to Consuela Coates-Beaufort, Elaine Auritt, Joseph Witkowski, and Bennett Ostroff, for their typing and patience in dealing with my too-frequent computer queries. A special note of thanks is reserved for Stephanie Warakomski, who endured my solitary, financially draining passion for a historical investigation of events that occurred almost a half century ago. Her patience and understanding are much appreciated.

I thank my many friends who encouraged me and lifted my occasionally flagging spirits as the months and years went by with no sure sign that the mystery surrounding the Holmesburg medical experiments would ever be revealed.

I extend my deepest thanks to the scores of individuals who consented to be interviewed—most of whom are listed below and many of whom were pressed to answer questions on several occasions—the historians, bioethicists, physicians, medical staff, and prison personnel.

Finally, I salute the courage, the fortitude, and the stories of the former inmates of Holmesburg Prison.

Notes

Introduction

1. In conversation with John Reeves, September 1971.
2. Ibid.
3. In conversation with George Washford (pseudonym), September 1971.
4. Interviews with Johnnie Williams, May 19, 1994, and James Sheffer, October 1994.
5. David J. Rothman, *Strangers at the Bedside* (New York: Basic Books, 1991).
6. Interview with Arthur Caplan.
7. George J. Annas and Michael A. Grodin, eds., *The Nazi Doctors and the Nuremberg Code* (New York: Oxford University Press, 1992).
8. Annas and Grodin, *The Nazi Doctors,* p. 228.
9. Senator Ted Kennedy, *Hearings on Human Experimentation,* part 3, March 7, 1973, p. 841.
10. Annas and Grodin, *The Nazi Doctors,* referring to *Tribunals of War Criminals before the Nuremberg Military Tribunals,* vol. 2, p. 181.
11. Eileen Welsome, "Plutonium Experiment," *Albuquerque Tribune,* November 15–17, 1993.
12. James H. Jones, *Bad Blood* (New York: Free Press, 1993).
13. Chip Brown, "The Science Club Serves Its Country," *Esquire* (December 1994), p. 122.
14. Allen Buchanan, "The Controversy over Retrospective Moral Judgment," *Kennedy Institute of Ethics Journal* 6, 3 (September 1996), p. 245.
15. Final Report, Advisory Committee on Human Radiation Experiments (Washington, D.C.: U.S. Government Printing Office, October 1995), p. 208.
16. Jay Katz, "Abuse of Human Beings for the Sake of Science," *When Medicine Went Mad* (Totowa, N.J.: Humana Press, 1992), p. 257.
17. M. H. Pappworth, *Human Guinea Pigs* (Boston: Beacon Press, 1967), p. 27.
18. Interview with Milton Cahn, February 8, 1996.
19. Interviews with A. Bernard Ackerman, beginning February 1, 1996–July 25, 1997.
20. Adolph Katz, "Prisoners Volunteer to Save Lives," *Philadelphia Bulletin,* February 27, 1966.

A Note on Sources

1. In order to protect the identities of the former and current prisoners with whom I spoke, unless express written permission was given to use their real names, I have used pseudonyms to conceal their identities. This designation is noted in the bibliography.
2. Documents obtained through the Freedom of Information Act from these government agencies will be abbreviated as follows:

Food and Drug Administration = F.O.I.A., FDA Documents
Central Intelligence Agency = F.O.I.A., CIA Documents
Department of Energy = F.O.I.A., DOE Documents
Department of the Army = F.O.I.A., Army Documents
Environmental Protection Agency = F.O.I.A., EPA Documents
U.S. Attorney General Office = F.O.I.A., USAGO Documents

Chapter One

1. Interviews with Al Zabala, March 16, 1994; April 27, 1994; November 3, 1994.
2. Interviews with Al Zabala.
3. Interview with Alex Gougnin, October 2, 1994.
4. William Robb, letter to the author, undated correspondence.
5. William Robb, correspondence.
6. Interview with Withers Ponton, April 28, 1994.
7. Interview with Ron Keenan, October 21, 1994.
8. Interview with Billy Allison, April 28, 1994.
9. Interview with James Kinslow, March 31, 1994.
10. Interview with Joseph Dade, April 27, 1994.
11. Interview with Hank Brame, March 3, 1994.
12. Daniel C. Martin, John D. Arnold, T. F. Zimmerman, and Robert Rickart, "Human Subjects in Clinical Research: A Report of Three Studies," *New England Journal of Medicine* 279, 26 (December 26, 1968).
13. William Robb, correspondence.
14. Interview with William Robb.
15. Interview with Ron Keenan.
16. Interview with Thomas Sims, May 3, 1994.
17. Interview with Tom McGevren, September 26, 1994.
18. Interview with Alvin Bronstein, June 22, 1994.
19. Interview with Sigmund Weitzman, May 10, 1994.
20. Interview with Roy Williams, May 11, 1994.
21. Interview with Sigmund Weitzman.
22. Interviews with William McCafferty, April 28, 1994 and November 3, 1994.
23. Interviews with William McCafferty.
24. Interviews with William McCafferty.
25. "Poison Ivy Picker of Pennypack Park," *Life* (September 1955).

26. Interviews with William McCafferty.
27. Interviews with William McCafferty.
28. Herbert Goldschmidt and Albert M. Kligman, "Experimental Inoculation of Humans with Ectodermotropic Viruses," *Journal of Investigative Dermatology* 31, 3 (September 1958): 175.
29. Christopher M. Papa and Albert M. Kligman, "The Behavior of Melanocytes in Inflammation," *Journal of Investigative Dermatology* 45, 6 (June 1965).
30. Interview with William McCafferty.
31. Interview with Leodus Jones, May 18, 1994.
32. Interview with Matthew Epps, April 28, 1994.
33. Interview with Matthew Epps.
34. Interview with Jay Biose.
35. Interview with Albert Levitt.
36. Interview with Priscilla Becroft, November 24, 1994.
37. Interview with Tom Shouler, June 14, 1997.
38. Interview with Scott Willson, December 1994.
39. Interview with Alex Gougnin, May 21, 1994.
40. Interview with Rick Mancini, April 28, 1994.
41. Interview with George Porter, June 1, 1994.
42. Interview with Andy Hollick, May 18, 1994.
43. Interview with James Lewis, July 7, 1994.
44. Jessica Mitford, "Experiments Behind Bars," *Atlantic Monthly* (January 1973); Robert E. Hodges and William B. Bean, "The Uses of Prisoners for Medical Research," *Journal of the American Medical Association* 202, 6 (November 6, 1967): 177; John D. Arnold, Daniel C. Martin, and Sarah E. Boyer, "A Study of One Prison Population and Its Responses to Medical Research," *Annals of the New York Academy of Sciences* 169 (January 21, 1970): 463; Excerpts appear in Jay Katz, *Experiments with Human Beings* (Russell Sage Foundation: New York, 1972), p. 1020.
45. Arnold et al. "A Study of One Prison Population." Also John C. McDonald, "Why Prisoners Volunteer To Be Experimental Subjects," *Journal of the American Medical Association* 202, 6 (1967): 175.
46. Interview with Billy Allison.
47. Interviews with Al Zabala.
48. Interview with Darren Sellner, September 20, 1994.
49. Interview with Fred Foxworth, June 7, 1994.
50. Interview with Jack Lopinson, March 14, 1994.
51. Interview with Hank Brame.
52. Interview with Al Butler, May 26, 1994.
53. Interview with Ron Keenan.
54. Interview with Al Butler.
55. Interview with Allan Lawson, June 14, 1994.
56. Interview with Raymond Crawford, April 28, 1994.
57. Interview with Simon Khaadim Ahad, April 28, 1994.
58. Interviews with Al Zabala.
59. Interview with Thomas Sims.

60. Interview with Withers Ponton.
61. Interview with Ron Keenan.
62. Interview with Alex Gougnin.
63. Interviews with Edmund Lyons, April 6, 1994 and December 15, 1994.
64. Interview with Sigmund Weitzman.

Chapter Two

1. "Philadelphia's New Prison," *Philadelphia Bulletin*, January 26, 1896.
2. John F. Morrison, "Reporter Called Holmesburg Prison 'Abhorrent' at its Opening in 1896," *Philadelphia Bulletin*, July 6, 1896.
3. "Trade School Seen as Convict's Need," *Philadelphia Bulletin*, October 8, 1923.
4. "Holmesburg Men Found Too Tough," *Philadelphia Bulletin*, March 20, 1929.
5. "Man Facing Loss of Feet Depicts Holmesburg Horror," *Philadelphia Bulletin*, February 22, 1929.
6. "Prisoners Beaten on Sorber's Order," *Philadelphia Bulletin*, February 26, 1929.
7. "Earle Bares Secret Device for Holmesburg Torture," *Philadelphia Bulletin*, August 31, 1938.
8. Interview with Leon Kneebone, January 22, 1996.
9. Albert M. Kligman, "The Handbook Of Mushroom Culture," *Science Press* (1942).
10. Albert M. Kligman, "Modern Spawn Making," *Science Press* (1941).
11. Interview with Leon Kneebone.
12. Lucinda Fleeson, "Saving Face," *Philadelphia Inquirer Sunday Magazine*, April 10, 1988, p. 16.
13. Interview with Beatrice Troyan, November 14, 1996.
14. A. M. Kligman, D. M. Pillsbury, and H. Mescon, "Improved Technique for Diagnosing Ringworm Infections and Moniliasis," *Journal of the American Medical Association* (August 25, 1951): 1563; A. M. Kligman, H. Mescon, and E. D. DeLamater, "The Hotchkiss-McManus Stain for the Histopathic Diagnosis of Fungus Disease," *American Journal of Clinical Pathology* 21, 86 (January 1951); A. M. Kligman, "Application of Potassium Hydroxide to the Skin as an Aid in Direct Examination of Scales for Fungi," *Archives of Dermatology & Syphiology* 63, 252 (February 1951).
15. Albert M. Kligman and W. Ward Anderson, "Evaluation of Current Methods for the Local Treatment of Tinea Capitis," *Journal of Investigative Dermatology*, 16 (March, 1951): 160.
16. Albert M. Kligman, "The Pathogenesis of Tinea Capitis Due to Microsporum Audouini and Microsporum Canis," *Journal of Investigative Dermatology* 18, 3, (March 1952): 231.
17. Frederick Deforest Weidman, "Discussion" of "The Pathogenesis of Tinea Capitis," *Journal of Investigative Dermatology* 18, 3, (March 1952): 246.
18. Donald M. Pillsbury, "Dr. Frederick Deforest Weidman," *Journal of Investigative Dermatology* 18, 3, (March 1952): 169.

19. Interview with Margaret Grey Wood, February 17, 1997.

20. Ibid.

21. Application for research grant, January 26, 1956. F.O.I.A., FDA Documents.

22. "Pathologic Reactions of the Fingernails Including Fungus Infections," p. 4.

23. Application for research grant. F.O.I.A., FDA Documents.

24. Interview with Dr. Albert M. Kligman, January 10, 1995.

25. Herman Beerman and Gerald Lazarus, *The Tradition of Excellence: Dermatology at the University of Pennsylvania* 1870–1985 (University of Pennsylvania Press, 1986), p. 132.

26. Adolph Katz, "Prisoners Volunteer To Save Lives," *Philadelphia Bulletin*, February 27, 1966.

27. Beerman and Lazarus, *Tradition of Excellence*, p. 132.

28. Interview with Dr. Albert M. Kligman.

29. Burton Chardak, "Prisoners Aid Research, 75% Here Act as Medical Guinea Pigs," *Philadelphia Bulletin*, September 18, 1960.

30. Katz, "Prisoners Volunteer To Save Lives."

31. Ibid.

32. Ibid.

33. Herbert Goldschmidt and Albert M. Kligman, "Experimental Inoculation of Humans with Ectodermotropic Viruses," *Journal of Investigative Dermatology*, 31, 3 (September 1958): 175

34. John S. Strauss and Albert M. Kligman, "Experimental Study of Tinea Pedis and Onychomycosis of the Foot," *Archives of Dermatology* 76 (1957): 70.

35. Howard I. Maibach and Albert M. Kligman, "The Biology of Experimental Human Cutaneous Moniliasis," *Archives of Dermatology*, 85 (1962): 233.

36. Gurmohan Singh, Richard R. Marples, and Albert M. Kligman, "Experimental Aureus Infection in Humans," *Journal of Investigative Dermatology*, 57, 3 (1971): 149.

37. Alfredo Rebora, Richard R. Marples, and Albert M. Kligman, "Experimental Infection with Candida Albicans," *Archives of Dermatology*, 108 (July 1973): 69.

38. Christopher M. Papa and Albert M. Kligman, "The Behavior of Melanocytes," *Journal of Investigative Dermatology*, 45, 6 (1965): 465.

39. Albert M. Kligman and Reinhard Briet, "The Identification of Phototoxic Drugs by Human Assay," *Journal of Investigative Dermatology*, 51, 2 (1968): 90.

40. Isaac Willis and Albert M. Kligman, "Photocontact Allergic Reactions," *Archives of Dermatology*, 100 (November 1969): 535.

41. Interview with Calvin Triol, October 8, 1994.

42. Interview with Edmund Lyons, April 4, 1994.

43. Interview with Alan Katz, October 7, 1994.

44. Interview with Clarence Livingood, March 20, 1996.

45. Interview with Walter Shelley, January 22, 1996.

46. Interview with Frederick Urbach, February 7, 1996.

47. Interview with Rudolph Baer, February 5, 1996.

48. Interview with Isaac Willis, February 2, 1996.
49. Interview with Paul Gross, January 22, 1996.
50. Interview with A. Bernard Ackerman, February 1, 1996.
51. Lucinda Fleeson, "Saving Face," *Philadelphia Inquirer Sunday Magazine,* April 10, 1988, p. 16.
52. Interview with Beatrice Troyan.
53. Interview with Alan Katz.
54. Interview with Alex Gougnin, June 21, 1994.
55. Interview with Al Butler, May 26, 1994.
56. Interview with Calvin Triol.
57. Interview with Tom Maeder, January 18, 1995.
58. Interview with Alan B. Lisook, January 13, 1995.
59. Interview with Dr. Milton Cahn, February 8, 1996.
60. Ibid.
61. Interview with Burt Cahn, February 8, 1996.
62. Interview with Milton Cahn.
63. Ibid.
64. Ann Selby, "Holmesburg Convicts Aid Medical Research," *Philadelphia Inquirer,* September 22, 1963.
65. Chardak, "Prisoners Aid Research."
66. Katz, "Prisoners Volunteer To Save Lives."
67. Chardak, "Prisoners Aid Research."
68. "100 Volunteers Will Do Time In Prison 'Climate Chamber,'" *Philadelphia Bulletin,* October 10, 1962.
69. Selby, "Holmesburg Convicts Aid Medical Research."
70. Interview with Beatrice Troyan.
71. Albert M. Kligman, letter to undisclosed, January 17, 1964. F.O.I.A., FDA Documents.
72. Undisclosed, letter to Albert M. Kligman, June 10, 1963.
73. Albert M. Kligman, letter and protocol to undisclosed, June 13, 1963.
74. Undisclosed, letter to Albert M. Kligman, June 18, 1963.
75. Undisclosed, letter to Albert M. Kligman, October 3, 1963.
76. Albert M. Kligman, letter to undisclosed, October 18, 1963.
77. Undisclosed, letter to Albert M. Kligman, October 21, 1963.
78. Undisclosed, letter to Albert M. Kligman, October 23, 1963.
79. Albert M. Kligman, letter to undisclosed, October 29, 1963.
80. Albert M. Kligman, letter to undisclosed, January 17, 1964.
81. Undisclosed, letter to Albert M. Kligman, January 22, 1964.
82. Albert M. Kligman, letter to undisclosed, February 4, 1964. F.O.I.A., FDA Documents.
83. R. J. Reynolds Tobacco Company, "Statement on Tryptophan Study in mid-1960s," January 13, 1997.
84. Ibid.
85. Christopher M. Papa and Albert M. Kligman, "Stimulation of Hair Growth by Topical Application of Androgens," *Journal of the American Medical Association* 191, 7 (February 15, 1965): 521.

86. "Baldness Breakthrough," Editorial in *Journal of the American Medical Association*, 191, 7 (February 15, 1965).
87. Beerman and Lazarus, *The Tradition of Excellence*, p. 132.
88. Albert M. Kligman, "Pathologic Dynamics of Human Hair Loss," *Archives of Dermatology* 83 (February 1961): 175.
89. Albert M. Kligman and Reinhard Breit, "The Identification of Phototoxic Drugs," *Journal of Investigative Dermatology* 51, 2 (1968): 90.
90. Albert M. Kligman, "Plastic Band-Aids for Patch Testing," *Archives of Dermatology* 75 (May 1957): 739.
91. James E. Fulton, Jr., Gerd Plewig and Albert M. Kligman, "Effect of Chocolate on Acne Vulgaris," *Journal of the American Medical Association* 210, 11 (December 15, 1969): 2071.
92. Interview with Alexander Capron, September 30, 1994.
93. Interview with Calvin Triol.
94. Gary Brooten, "FDA Ban on Drug Tests by U. of P. Specialist Imperils Research Program at Holmesburg Prison," *Philadelphia Sunday Bulletin*, July 31, 1966, p. 27.
95. A. Harris Kenyon, memorandum to Directors of Districts, July 19, 1966. F.O.I.A., FDA Documents.
96. Interview with Alan B. Lisook, January 19, 1996.
97. Interview with Frances O. Kelsey, January 12, 1995.
98. David M. Cleary, "U. of P. Doctor is Reinstated as Drug Tester by U.S. Agency," *Philadelphia Bulletin*, August 25, 1966.
99. Brooten, "FDA Ban."
100. Albert M. Kligman, "Topical Pharmacology and Toxicology of Dimethyl Sulfoxide," Part I, *Journal of the American Medical Association* 193, 10 (September 6, 1965).
101. Interview with Alan B. Lisook.
102. W. B. Rankin, letter to various drug companies, July 19, 1966. F.O.I.A., FDA Documents.
103. Brooten, "FDA Ban."
104. Ibid.
105. Ibid.
106. Ibid.
107. "Investigating the Investigator," *Time* (August 5, 1966).
108. Brooten, "FDA Ban."
109. W. B. Rankin, letter to variety of drug companies, August 19, 1966. F.O.I.A., FDA Documents.
110. Interview with Frances Kelsey.
111. Interview with Alan Lisook.
112. Interview with Solomon McBride, December 8, 1994.
113. Albert M. Kligman, "Dimethyl Sulfoxide—A Correction," *Journal of the American Medical Association* 197, 13 (September 26, 1966): 161.
114. Jennifer Newman, "Wrinkle Warrior," *American Health* (September 1992): 19.
115. Interview with Alan Lisook.
116. Frances O. Kelsey, memorandum to Herbert L. Ley, March 1, 1967. F.O.I.A., FDA Documents.

117. Robert J. Robinson, memorandum to Office of the Commissioner, June 30, 1966. F.O.I.A., FDA Documents.
118. Harold C. Anderson, "Evaluation of Tolerance Study and Meeting," undated. F.O.I.A., FDA Documents.
119. Harold C. Anderson, memorandum of conference, May 19, 1966. F.O.I.A., FDA Documents.
120. W. B. Rankin, memorandum of conference, July 22, 1966. F.O.I.A., FDA Documents.
121. Donald M. Pillsbury, letter to W. B. Rankin, July 26, 1966. F.O.I.A., FDA Documents.
122. Harold C. Anderson, memorandum to Robert J. Robinson, August 4, 1966. F.O.I.A., FDA Documents.
123. Ibid.
124. Donald M. Pillsbury, letter to W. B. Rankin, August 12, 1966. F.O.I.A., FDA Documents.
125. Robert J. Robinson, memorandum to W. B. Rankin, August 15, 1966; W. B. Rankin, handwritten note on memorandum, August 15, 1966. F.O.I.A., FDA Documents.
126. Donald M. Pillsbury, letter to W. B. Rankin, October 17, 1966. F.O.I.A., FDA Documents.
127. Donald M. Pillsbury, letter to W. B. Rankin, November 29, 1966. F.O.I.A., FDA Documents.
128. Interviews with Calvin Triol.
129. Interviews with Edward Lyons, April 6, 1994, and December 15, 1994.
130. Interviews with Calvin Triol.
131. Interview with Alan Katz.
132. Interview with Solomon McBride.
133. "Final Report of the Advisory Committee on Human Radiation Experiments," October, 1995.
134. Interview with Solomon McBride.
135. Interview with Alan Katz.
136. Interview with Melvin Heller, September 20, 1994.
137. Melvin S. Heller, "Problems and Prospects in the Use of Prison Inmates for Medical Experiments," *The Prison Journal* 57, 1 (Spring 1967): 21.
138. Interview with Arthur Boxer, November 1994.
139. Interview with Edward Guy, October 1994.
140. Interview with Aron Start, May 1994.
141. Interview with Alvin Bronstein, June 22, 1994.
142. Interviews with Calvin Triol.
143. Interview with Solomon McBride.
144. Interview with Albert M. Kligman, January 10, 1995.
145. Beerman and Lazarus, *The Tradition of Excellence*, p. 132.
146. Jessica Mitford, *Kind and Usual Punishment* (New York: Knopf, 1973).
147. Interview with Jessica Mitford, October 23, 1995.

Chapter Three

1. George J. Annas and Michael A. Grodin, eds., *The Nazi Doctors and the Nuremberg Code* (New York: Oxford University Press, 1992), p. 99.
2. Ibid., p. 66.
3. Ibid., p. 137.
4. *Journal of Zoophily* 16 (1907): 94.
5. M. H. Pappworth, *Human Guinea Pigs* (Boston: Beacon Press, 1967), p. 61.
6. Richard P. Strong, "Vaccination Against Plague," *Philippine Journal of Science* 181: 186; and Eli Cherin, "Richard Pearson Strong and the Iatrogenic Plague Disaster in Bilibid Prison, Manila, 1906," *Reviews of Infectious Diseases* 11, 6, (November 1989): 996.
7. Ibid.
8. *Journal of Zoophily* 16 (1907): 94.
9. Ibid.
10. Annas and Grodin, *The Nazi Doctors and the Nuremberg Code*, p. 97.
11. Elizabeth W. Etheridge, *The Butterfly Caste* (Westport, CT: Greenwood Publishing, 1972), p. 7.
12. Ibid.
13. Ibid., p. 96.
14. L. L. Stanley, "An Analysis of One Thousand Testicular Substance Implantations," *Endocrinology* 6 (1922): 787; Susan E. Lederer, *Subjected to Science* (Baltimore: Johns Hopkins University Press, 1995), p. 111.
15. Stanley, "An Analysis" p. 788.
16. "Felons Gather for Test," *New York Times*, March 26, 1934.
17. Robert R. Logan, ed. "Criminal Guinea Pigs" The Starry Cross, Vol. 43, No. 2 (Philadelphia: American Antivivisection Society:1935), p. 19.
18. S. H. Besley, "Heart at Death," *Life* (November 7, 1938): 20.
19. Don Wharton, "Prisoners Who Volunteer, Blood, Flesh and Their Lives," *The American Mercury* 79 (1954): 53.
20. Ibid., p. 51.
21. John L. O'Hara, "The Most Unforgettable Character I've Met," *Reader's Digest* 52 (May 1948): 32.
22. Nathan Leopold, *Life Plus 99 years* (Garden City, N.Y.: Doubleday, 1958).
23. *Life* (June 4, 1945): 43.
24. *New York Times*, March 5, 1945, p. 1.
25. Pappworth, *Human Guinea Pigs*, p. 62.
26. Leopold, *Life Plus 99 years*; and "Guinea Pigs Pardoned," *New York Times*, December 31, 1949.
27. Jacob George, "Atlanta's Malaria Project," *Atlantian* 6, 3 (January–March 1946): 14.
28. Ibid., p. 43.
29. Ibid.
30. "Federal Prisons Year End Review," 1944, p. 22.
31. "Federal Prisons Year End Review," 1946, p. 31.
32. "Federal Prisons Year End Review," 1949, p. 34.

33. David J. Rothman, "Henry Beecher Revisited," *New England Journal of Medicine* 317, 19 (November 7, 1987).
34. *Abridged Transcripts of the Nuremberg Medical Trial*, Vol. 1, p. 27.
35. David J. Rothman, *Strangers at the Bedside* (New York: Basic Books, 1991), p. 51.
36. Ibid., p. 53.
37. *United States v. Karl Brandt et al. Trials of War Criminals before the Nuremberg Military Tribunals under Control Council Law*, no. 10, June 13, 1947, A-MJ-23-2 Gross (Brown) Court I, p. 9171.
38. Ibid., p. 9141.
39. "Ethics Governing the Services of Prisoners as Subjects in Medical Experiments: Report of a Committee Appointed by Governor Dwight H. Green of Illinois," *Journal of the American Medical Association* 136 (February 14, 1948): 457.
40. "Convict Joins Own Blood Stream to That of Girl Dying of Cancer," *New York Times*, June 4, 1949, p. 1.
41. "Convict's Blood Gift Fails To Save Girl, 8," *New York Times*, June 8, 1949, p. 1.
42. "Blood Exchanger Named," *New York Times*, June 23, 1949.
43. "Sing Sing Lifer Freed By Dewey," *New York Times*, December 23, 1949, p. 1.
44. "Pardoned Lifer Returns to Son," *New York Times*, December 24, 1949.
45. Ludwig Gross, Letter to the Editor, *New York Times*, December 31, 1949.
46. George Annas, "The Nuremberg Code in U.S. Courts," in *The Nazi Doctors and the Nuremberg Code*, p. 217.
47. "Federal Prisons Year End Review," 1953, p. 31-33.
48. Ibid.
49. Ibid.
50. Ibid.
51. Ibid.
52. "Vaccine Is Called Effective for Cold Type Infections," *New York Times*, November 4, 1955, p. 2.
53. "New Live Virus Polio Vaccine, Taken Orally, to Get Mass Test," *New York Times*, October 7, 1956.
54. "Syphilis Vaccine Gains," *New York Times*, December 9, 1954.
55. "Convicts Aiding Science," *New York Times*, July 20, 1953.
56. Morris Kaplan, "Tests on Convicts Curb Vaccine Ills," *New York Times*, October 11, 1947.
57. "Women Prisoners Aid Jaundice Test," *New York Times*, September 4, 1950.
58. W. J. H. Butterfield, letter to Richard W. Copelan, October 30, 1951. The Archives Department of Thompkins-McCaw Library of the Medical College of Virginia, Richmond, Virginia. [hereafter TMLMCV].
59. W. J. H. Butterfield, letter to W. F. Smyth, October 30, 1951. TMLMCV.
60. W. F. Smyth, Jr., letter to Medical College of Virginia, December 19, 1951. TMLMCV.
61. Everett Idris Evans, letter to W. F. Smyth, January 18, 1952. TMLMCV.
62. W. J. H. Butterfield, memorandum on "Observation on Volunteers from Penitentiary," 1951, p. 5. TMLMCV.
63. Undisclosed name, letter to B. W. Haynes, May 21, 1955. TMLMCV.

64. Robert E. Hodges and William B. Bean, "The Use of Prisoners for Medical Research," *Journal of the American Medical Association* 202, 6 (November 6, 1967): 543-75.
65. "Cancer By the Needle," *Newsweek* (June 4, 1956): 67.
66. "Cancer Volunteers" *Time* 69 (February 25, 1957): 46.
67. Ruth Faden and Tom Beauchamp, *A History and Theory of Informed Consent* (New York: Oxford University Press, 1986).
68. Interview with Chester Southam, June 28, 1996.
69. Nicholas Horrock, "Records Show CIA Tested LSD on Sex-Psychopaths" *New York Times*, August 5, 1977, p. A10
70. "Prison Volunteers Test Vaccine for Tularemia," *Science News Letter* (June 22, 1957): 386.
71. Department of Health and Human Services, 45 CFR: part 46, *Federal Register* 46, 16, (January 26, 1981): 8389; Food and Drug Administration, 21 CFR: part 50, *Federal Register* 46, 17 (January 27, 1981): 8951.
72. Interview with Gerald Wachs, January 7, 1997.
73. Walter Rugaber, "Prison Drug and Plasma Projects Leave Fatal Trail," *New York Times*, July 29, 1969, p. 1.
74. Ibid.
75. Ibid.
76. Ibid.
77. Ibid.
78. Walter Sullivan, "Scientist Reports Isolating 2 Strains of Hepatitis," *New York Times*, June 29, 1961, and "Vaccination Reported for Infectious Hepatitis," *New York Times*, May 5, 1961.
79. Ibid.
80. Marjorie Hunter, "Drug Is Reported to Avert Malaria," *New York Times*, November 2, 1962, p. 33.
81. Howard A. Rusk, "Drugs and Prisoners," *New York Times*, November 11, 1962, p. 74.
82. "Prisoners Help Test Drug for Malaria," *New York Times*, March 16, 1966.
83. Harold M. Schmeck, Jr., "Scientists Trace a Sneeze's Spread," *New York Times*, April 14, 1966, p. 72.
84. Harold M. Schmeck, Jr., "Sprayed Vaccine for Flu Called Better Than Shots," *New York Times*, May 6, 1968.
85. Jane E. Brody, "Vitamin C Study Rebuts Pauling," *New York Times*, November 28, 1971.
86. Gene I. Maeroff, "Influenza Tests Hint Better Drug," *New York Times*, August 13, 1972.
87. Adams and Cowan, "The Human Guinea Pig," p. 20.
88. "Drug Tests Behind Bars," *Business Week* (June 27, 1964): 62.
89. Jessica Mitford, "Experiments Behind Bars: Doctors, Drug Companies, and Prisoners," *Atlantic Monthly* (January 1973): 69.
90. Ibid.
91. Pat Duffy, Jr., "Drug Testing in Prisons: The View from Inside," in D. Basson, Rachel E. Lipson, Doreen L. Ganos, eds., *Troubling Problems in*

Medical Ethics (New York: Alan R. Liss, 1981), p. 79.

92. Jessica Mitford, "Experiments Behind Bars," and *Kind and Unusual Punishment* (New York: Vintage Books, 1974), p. 172.

93. Ibid.

94. Gary Lee, "The Lifelong Harm to Radiation's Human Guinea Pigs," *Washington Post,* National Weekly Edition, November 28, 1994, p. 33.

95. Ibid.

96. Ibid.

97. Ibid.

98. Ibid.

99. Dr. John L. Sever and Dr. Jerome E. Kurent, Project Protocol, "Development of Immune Responses to Rubeola and Rubella Vaccines."

100. "Outline of Information for Potential Volunteers Metabolic Service," U.S. Public Health Service Hospital, San Francisco, California, November 14, 1969.

101. Mitford, *Kind and Usual Punishment,* p. 152.

102. Senate Committee on Labor and Public Welfare, Subcommittee on Health, Quality of Health Care—Human Experimentation, 1973: Hearings on S.974, S.878, and S. J. Res. 71, 93rd Cong., March 7, 1973.

103. "Jailed Guinea Pigs," editorial in *New York Times,* October 23, 1974.

104. "Prison Official in Illinois Halts Malaria Research on Inmates," *New York Times,* April 28, 1974.

105. H. R. 16160, 93rd Cong., 2nd sess., July 29, 1974.

106. H. R. 3603, 94th Cong., 1st sess., February 24, 1975.

107. Irving Gilchrist, "Black Balling Tesimony," *Medical Research on Prisoners Clearinghouse to End Medical Experimentation* 4 (September 1975).

108. Prison Inmates in Medical Research: Hearings on H. R. 3606, 94th Cong. 1st. sess, September 29, 1975, p. 1.

109. Hearings before the Subcommittee on Health of the Committee on Labor and Public Welfare—U.S. Senate, 93rd Cong., March 7–8, 1973, p. 866.

110. Sam Ervin, Jr., letter to Norman Carlson, January 7, 1974.

111. Harold R. Tyler, Jr., and Norman A. Carlson, "H.R. 3603—Use of Federal Prisoners in Medical Research Projects," October 2, 1975.

112. Norman A. Carlson, letter to deputy attorney general on medical experimentation, March 2, 1976.

113. Victor Cohn, "Medical Research on Prisoners, Poor Defended, Hit."

114. Victor Cohn, "Inmates Oppose Experiment Halt," *Washington Post,* November 16, 1975.

115. "Report and Recommendations: Research Involving Prisoners," *The National Commission for the Protection of Human Subjects of Biomedical and Behavioral Research* (Washington, D.C.: DHEW, 1976), p. 8.

116. Carlson, letter to deputy attorney general.

117. "Government to Ban Medical Research on Federal Inmates," *New York Times,* March 2, 1976.

118. Rothman, *Strangers at the Bedside.*

119. Harold M. Schmeck, Jr., "Curbs on Biomedical Tests on Humans Proposed by Panels at Minority Parley," *New York Times,* January 9, 1976.

120. *Code of Federal Regulations* 21, part 50, 44, "Restrictions on Clinical Investigations Involving Prisoners."

Chapter Four

1. Interviews with Johnnie Williams, May 19, 1994; July 20, 1994; and October 21, 1994.
2. Interviews with James Ketchum, February 15, 1995; March 1, 1995; and April 10, 1995.
3. Committee on Toxicology, *Possible Long-Term Health Effects of Short-Term Exposure to Chemical Agents* (Washington, D.C.: National Academy Press, 1982), p. 1.
4. Ibid., introduction.
5. Ibid.
6. Ibid.
7. James Ketchum and Frederick Sidell, "Incapacitating Compounds—Draft Print," p. 12.
8. Report of the Inspector General, Department of the Army, 1975. F.O.I.A. Army Documents.
9. James S. Ketchum, David Kitzes, and Herbert Copelan, "EA 3167: Effects in Man," Edgewood Arsenal, Maryland, January, 1975.
10. Interview with Lawrence Byrne, December 7, 1994.
11. Ketchum, Kitzes, and Copelan, "EA 3167," p. 11.
12. CIA memorandum, Review of "EA 3167" Study, June 23, 1970. F.O.I.A., CIA Documents.
13. Ketchum, Kitzes, and Copelan, "EA 3167," p. 11.
14. Report of the Inspector General, Department of the Army, 1975, p. 157. F.O.I.A., Army Documents.
15. Ibid., p. 158.
16. Ibid., p. 163.
17. Ibid., p. 166.
18. Ibid., p. 158.
19. Ibid., p. 166.
20. Interviews with James Ketchum.
21. Aaron Epstein, "At Holmesburg, 320 Guinea Pigs," *Philadelphia Inquirer,* November 25, 1979.
22. Interview with James Ketchum.
23. Interview with Frederick Sidell, December 15, 1994.
24. Interviews with James Ketchum.
25. Interview with Alan Katz, October 7, 1994.
26. Comments about legal concerns arose in conversations with John Chichi, Calvin Triol, Alan Katz, Milton Cahn, Paul Gross, and A. Bernard Ackerman, among others.
27. Interview with James Ketchum.
28. Interview with James Ketchum.
29. Herbert W. Copelan, Report Number VII, ID 50 of Agent 926 Final Report, July 6, 1970.

30. John Marks, *The Search for the Manchurian Candidate* (New York: W. W. Norton, 1979) p. 33. (DOE)

31. CIA memorandum for the record, Trip Report/ Edgewood Arsenal, February 12, 1975. (CIA)

32. U. S. Senate Committee, Joint Hearing before the Select Committee on Health and Scientific Research of the Committee of Human Resources, *CIA Program on Research in Behavioral Modification*, 95th Cong., August 3, 1977, p. 5.

33. Marks, *Search for the Manchurian Candidate*, p. 63.

34. CIA memorandum, Influencing Human Behavior, undated. (CIA)

35. CIA memorandum for Inspector General, May 6, 1974, p. 3. (CIA)

36. Marks, *Search for the Manchurian Candidate*, p. 33.

37. CIA memorandum, Follow-on Contract, March 24, 1969. (CIA)

38. Ibid.

39. Ibid., p.2.

40. CIA memorandum, Follow-on Contract, March 8, 1971. (CIA)

41. CIA document, Materials Analysis, undated. (CIA)

42. Ketchum, "EA-3167."

43. CIA, memorandum for Director of Research and Development, May 29, 1973. (CIA)

44. Interview with Frederick Sidell, February 6, 1996.

45. Project MKULTRA, The CIA's Program of Research in Behavioral Modification, Joint Hearing before the Select Committee on Intelligence, August 3, 1977, p. 32. (CIA)

46. CIA memorandum for Deputy Director for Science and Technology, October 19, 1978. (CIA)

47. H Block Log Book, Holmesburg Prison, April 30, 1968–May 7, 1969, p. 56.

48. Albert M. Kligman and Herbert W. Copelan, *Annual Report*, University of Pennsylvania Research Unit, May, 1967, p. 1. (Army)

49. Ibid., p. 2.

50. Ibid.

51. Christopher M. Papa and Albert M. Kligman, "The Behavior of Melanocytes in Inflammation," *Journal of Investigative Dermatology* 45, 6 (1965): 465. (Army)

52. Ibid.

53. A. M. Kligman, Holmesburg Prison Annual Report, March 31, 1966. (Army)

54. A. M. Kligman, Holmesburg Prison Monthly Progress Report, March 31, 1965. (Army)

55. Kligman, Holmesburg Prison Annual Report, 1966. (Army)

56. Herbert W. Copelan, Report Number V, "Med 50 of Agent 282," May 1967. (Army)

57. Herbert W. Copelan, Report Number I, "Med 50 of Agent 834," August 1968. (Army)

58. Herbert W. Copelan, Report Number IV, "Med 50 of Agent CAR 302,212," January 31, 1967. (Army)

59. Herbert W. Copelan and Albert M. Kligman, Report Number III, "Med 50 of Agent CAR 302,368," November 22, 1966. (Army)
60. Epstein, "At Holmesburg Prison, 320 Human Guinea Pigs."
61. Ibid.
62. Interviews with Johnnie Wlliams.

Chapter Five

1. Albert M Kligman, Application for By-Product Material License, August 26, 1963. (DOE)
2. "Final Report of the Advisory Committee on Human Radiation Experiments," October, 1995, p. 433.
3. Lee Davidson, "Did Secret Radiation Tests on Inmates Doom Offspring?" *Deseret News*, November 10, 1994, p. A1.
4. "Final Report," p. 434.
5. Ibid., p. 435.
6. Ibid., p. 421.
7. Ibid., p. 424.
8. Ibid., p. 424
9. Ibid., p. 425.
10. Ibid., p. 427.
11. Ibid., p. 428.
12. Ibid., p. 430.
13. Ibid., p. 431.
14. Gary Lee, "The Lifelong Harm to Radiation's Human Guinea Pigs," *Washington Post*, National Weekly Edition, November 28, 1994, p. 33.
15. Ibid., p.33.
16. Ibid., p. 34.
17. John S. Strauss and Albert M. Kligman, "Distribution of Skin Doses over Scalp in Therapy of Tinea Capitis with Superficial X-Rays," *Archives of Dermatology & Syphilology* 70, 1: 331.
18. Ibid., p. 335.
19. Ibid., p. 342.
20. Interview with John F. Wilson, March 3, 1997.
21.Kligman Application, 1963. (DOE)
22. Ibid.
23. Interview with Benjamin Calesnick, November 27, 1995.
24. John E. Bowyer, letter to Benjamin Calesnick, October 20, 1964. (DOE)
25. Benjamin Calesnick, letter to John E. Bowyer of U.S. Atomic Energy Commission, October 23, 1964. (DOE)
26. Kligman, Application, 1963. (DOE)
27. Arthur W. Wase, letter to U.S. Atomic Energy Commission, October 29, 1964. (DOE)
28. R. W. Rawson, Atomic Energy Commission Appraisal, September 24, 1963. (DOE)
29. John E. Bowyer, letter to A. M. Kligman, October 9, 1963. (DOE)

30. H. Earle Tucker, letter to John E. Bowyer, October 25, 1963. (DOE)
31. John E. Bowyer, U.S. Atomic Energy Commission By-Product Material License, January 8, 1964. (DOE)
32. John E. Bowyer, letter to Holmesburg Prison, attn.: A. M. Kligman, December 2, 1964. (DOE)
33. Albert M.Kligman, Application for By-Product Material License, July 27, 1965. (DOE)
34. Ibid. (DOE)
35. Kligman Application, 1965. (DOE)
36. Interview with Benjamin Calesnick. (DOE)
37. Albert M. Kligman, "Studies of Human Epidermal Turnover Time Using S^{35} Cystine and H^3 Thymidine and of Cutaneous Permeability Using C^{14} Testosterone and Corticosteroid," March 14, 1966. (DOE)
38. W. D. Armstrong, Atomic Energy Commission Appraisal, May 5, 1966. (DOE)
39. John A. D. Cooper, Atomic Energy Commission Appraisal, April 26, 1966. (DOE)
40. Reynold F. Brown, Atomic Energy Commission Appraisal, May 31, 1966. (DOE)
41. R. W. Rawson, Atomic Energy Commission Appraisal, March 31, 1966. (DOE)
42. Albert M. Kligman, Application for By-Product Material License, April 25, 1968. (DOE)
43. A. M. Kligman and Herbert W. Copelan, Holmesburg Prison Annual Report, May, 1967. (Army)
44. Interview with Paul Goldberg, November 13, 1995.
45. Interview with Issac Willis, February 6, 1996.
46. Interview with Benjamin Calesnick.

Chapter Six

1. Interviews with Alfonso Zabala, February 9–10, 1996.
2. Alfonso Zabala, letter to EPA, May 6, 1981. (EPA)
3. Aaron Epstein, "Human Guinea Pigs: Dioxin Tested at Holmesburg," *Philadelphia Inquirer*, January 11, 1981.
4. Ibid.
5. Verald Keith Rowe, testimony before EPA, November 13, 1980. (EPA)
6. Ibid.
7. Verald Keith Rowe, Dow Chemical Company memorandum, December 24, 1964. (EPA)
8. Ibid.
9. Verald Keith Rowe, Dow Chemical Company memorandum, March 4, 1965. (EPA)
10. Albert M. Kligman, letter to Verald Keith Rowe, March 2, 1965. (EPA)
11. Adele S. Allen (Secretary to Albert M. Kligman), letter to Verald Keith Rowe, March 10, 1965.

12. Verald Keith Rowe, letter to Albert M. Kligman, July 9, 1965. (EPA)
13. Albert M. Kligman, letter to Verald Keith Rowe, May 11, 1966. (EPA)
14. Ibid.
15. Interviews with Verald Keith Rowe, February 9, 1996; February 12; 1996, and April 17, 1994.
16. Kligman letter to Rowe, May 11, 1966. (EPA)
17. Rowe, testimony before EPA. (EPA)
18. Albert M. Kligman, letter to Verald Keith Rowe, June 22, 1966. (EPA)
19. Albert M. Kligman, letter to Verald Keith Rowe, January 23, 1968. (EPA)
20. Interviews with Verald Keith Rowe.
21. Interviews with Verald Keith Rowe.
22. Albert M. Kligman, letter to Verald Keith Rowe, January 23, 1968. (EPA)
23. Rowe, testimony before EPA. (EPA)
24. Ibid.
25. Interviews with Verald Keith Rowe.
26. Name withheld, letter to EPA, January 12, 1981. (EPA)
27. Name withheld, affidavit to EPA, February 4, 1981. (EPA)
28. "Agent Orange Tested on Convicts," *Detroit Free Press*, January 12, 1981. (EPA)
29. Name withheld, letter to EPA, January 23, 1986. (EPA)
30. Name withheld, letter to EPA, January 11, 1981. (EPA)
31. Epstein, "Human Guinea Pigs."
32. Aaron Epstein, "Inquiries Surface on Dioxin," *Philadelphia Inquirer*, January 25, 1981.
33. Interview with Sigmund Weitzman, August 1994.
34. Ibid.
35. Ibid.
36. Epstein, "Inquiries Surface."
37. Harold Jamison, "2 Men Scarred for Life by Prison Tests," *Philadelphia Tribune*, January 30, 1981.
38. Harold Jamison, "EPA Seeks 13 Used as Guinea Pigs in Tests," *Philadelphia Tribune*, January 27, 1981.
39. Johnnie Williams, "A Clear Case of Genocide," *Philadelphia Tribune*, January 23, 1981.
40. Harold Jamison, "Man Killed by Police was Used as Prison Guinea Pig," *Philadelphia Tribune*, January 23, 1981.
41. Van Kozak, EPA document, "TCDD Dosing of Prisoners," January 29, 1981. (EPA)
42. Ibid.
43. John W. Kliewer, EPA document, "TCDD Dosing of Prisoners," March 4, 1981. (EPA)
44. Donald Barnes, EPA document, "Summary of Holmesburg Prison Study," May 8, 1981.
45. Frank Davido, EPA document, Holmesburg Dioxin Testing, May 13, 1981. (EPA)
46. John W. Melone, Status of Action Plan for Holmesburg Prison, August 14, 1981. (EPA)

47. EPA memorandum, Status of Prisoner Test Subjects, Spring 1981. (EPA)
48. Frank L. Davido, rejection letter to Alfonso Zabala, June 22, 1981. (EPA)
49. Frank L. Davido, letter to Mr. Barnwell, January 12, 1982. (EPA)
50. Frank L. Davido, Holmesburg Prison memorandum, January 12, 1982. (EPA)
51. Interview with Frank Davido, February 20, 1996.
52. Frank L. Davido, letter to Alfonso Zabala, March 31, 1982. (EPA)
53. Frank L. Davido, letter and final report to Alfonso Zabala, July 22, 1982. (EPA)
54. Donald P. Morgan, letter to Bob Heath, May 25, 1982. (EPA)
55. William Robbins, "Dioxin tests conducted in 60s on 70 Philadelphia Inmates, Now Unknown," *New York Times*, July 17, 1983.
56. *Robert D. Crew, Bonnie C. Crew, Leodus Jones, George Askew, and Earl Charles Harris v. The Dow Chemical Company et al.*, United States District Court, Eastern District of Pennsylvania, no. 81-4824.
57. Jamison, "EPA Seeks 13 Used as Guinea Pigs."
58. Interview with Leodus Jones, May 18, 1994.
59. *William Smith v. Albert Kligman, Ivy Research, Solomon McBride, Trustees of University of Pennsylvania, Dow Chemical, Philadelphia Prisons and City of Philadelphia*, Court of Common Pleas, Philadelphia, January 1983.
60. Vernon Loeb, "Suit Settled over Alleged Dioxin Tests," *Philadelphia Inquirer*, December 4, 1986.
61. Ibid.
62. *James Walker and Shirley Walker v. Albert Kligman, Ivy Research Laboratories, Trustees of the University of Pennsylvania and the City of Philadelphia*, Court of Common Pleas, Philadelphia, September 1979.
63. Ray Holton, "Suit Filed in Drug Tests on Inmates," *Philadelphia Inquirer*, January 11, 1980.

Chapter Seven

1. Lou Antosh, "Medical Testing Lab Closed at Holmesburg," *Philadelphia Bulletin*, January 29, 1974.
2. Ibid.
3. Ibid.
4. David Cleary, "Kligman Admits Inaccuracy in Science Reporting," *Philadelphia Bulletin*, September 27, 1966.
5. Alan Davis, "Sexual Assaults in the Philadelphia Prison System and Sheriff's Vans," December 1968.
6. Ibid., p.761.
7. Ibid., p. 762.
8. Ibid., p.765.
9. Ibid., p. 766.
10. Ibid., P. 767.
11. Ibid., p. 768.

12. William B. Collins, "Lab Testing Program Tied to Prison Sex Corruptions," *Philadelphia Inquirer*, September 12, 1968.
13. "Chalfin Asks Pact on Medical Research on Prisoners," *Philadelphia Bulletin*, January 14, 1969.
14. Interview with Paul M. Chalfin, October 12, 1994.
15. Interview with Charles Mirarchi, June 28, 1994.
16. Interview with Artis Ray, September 1994.
17. Quality of Health Care—Human Experimentation, U.S. Senate Committee on Labor and Public Welfare, March 7–8, 1973.
18. Ibid. p. 822.
19. Ibid. p. 823.
20. Ibid., p. 824.
21. Ibid., p. 825.
22. Ibid., p. 826.
23. Ibid., p. 827.
24. Interview with Allan Lawson, June 14, 1994.
25. Interview with Mattie Humphrey, February 4, 1997.
26. Interview with Spencer Coxe, June 19, 1997.
27. David Rudovsky, Statement of American Civil Liberties Union, Greater Philadelphia Branch at Hearings On Medical Experimentation In State And Country Institutions, Pennsylvania Departments of Justice & Public Welfare, Harrisburg, Pennsylvania, June 21, 1973.
28. Interview with Marvin Wolfgang, September 1994
29. *Roach v. Kligman*, Civil Action No. 73-2428, April 30, 1976.
30. "Ex-Inmate Sues Lab and City over Research Test on Him," *Philadelphia Evening Bulletin*, October 26, 1973.
31. Interview with David Rudovsky, June, 1995.
32. Deposition of Albert M. Kligman, *Roach v. Kligman*, June 19, 1974.
33. Deposition of Herbert W. Copelan, *Roach v. Kligman*, July 30, 1974.
34. Deposition of Luther M. Mitchell, *Roach v. Kligman*, June 6, 1974.
35. Deposition of Albert M. Kligman.
36. "Consent to Participate in Medical Study," October 24, 1972.
37. Deposition of Albert M. Kligman.
38. Norman R. Ingraham, Jr. (University of Pennsylvania department of dermatology stationery), letter to Emily Stannard, November 30, 1950. Norman R. Ingraham, Jr. (Philadelphia department of public health stationery), letter to Emily Stannard, January 4, 1951. University of Pennsylvania Research Archives.
39. Interviews with Jack Hepp, Jr., July 26, 1995, and May 12, 1996.
40. Ruth Faden and Tom Beauchamp, *A History and Theory of Informed Consent* (Oxford University Press: New York: 1986), p. 208.
41. Deposition of Albert M. Kligman.
42. Louis G. Aytch Answers Plaintiff's First Interrogatories, *Roach v. Kligman*, July 16, 1974, and Affidavit, October 7, 1974.
43. Interview with Howard M. Rawnsley, September 27, 1994.
44. H. C. Maguire and A. M. Kligman, "Norwegian Scabies," *Archives of*

Dermatology 82 (1960): p. 62 and H. C. Maguire and A. M. Kligman, "Histopathology of Common Male Baldness," *Proceedings of XII Congress of Dermatology,* 1963, p. 1438.

45. Interview with Henry C. Maguire, December 17, 1996.
46. Interview with Seymour M. Johnson, Jr., September, 1994.
47. Interview with Cecil O. Smith, Jr., September 22, 1994.
48. Interview with Victor H. Carpenter, September 1994.
49. Interview with Allyn Sielaff, December 7, 1994.
50. Interview with Lucien Blackwell, October 24, 1996.

Chapter Eight

1. Advertisment © Ortho Pharmaceutical Corporation 1996. *Archives of Dermatology* 132 (July 1996): 757.
2. Beverly A. Pawson, "History of Retinoids," *Journal of the American Academy of Dermatology* 6, 4 (April 1982): 579.
3. Albert M. Kligman, Otto Mills, James J. Leyden, Paul Gross, Herbert B. Allen, and Robert I. Rudolph, "Oral Vitamin A in Acne Vulgaris," *International Journal of Dermatology* (May 1981): 278.
4. Jonathan V. Straumfjord, "Vitamin A: Its Effects on Acne," *Northwest Medicine* 42 (August 1943): 225.
5. C. Stuttgen, "Zur Lokalbehandlung von Keratosen mit Vitamin A Saure," *Dermatologica* 124 (February 1962): 78.
6. Interview with C. Stuttgen, December 20, 1996.
7. Interview with Philip Frost, February 26, 1996.
8. Stephen Fried, "Facing Up to Retin-A®," *Philadelphia Magazine,* April 1996, p. 104.
9. Interview with Gerd Plewig, May 22, 1996.
10. Interview with Chalmers E. Cornelius, III, November 25, 1996.
11. Interview with Joseph Witkowski, January 3, 1997.
12. Albert M. Kligman, James E. Fulton, Jr., and Gerd Plewig, "Topical Vitamin A Acid in Acne Vulgaris," *Archives of Dermatology* 99 (April 1969): 471.
13. Advertisement © Ortho Pharmaceutical Corporation 1995.
14. "New Acne Treatment Found by Researchers," *Philadelphia Bulletin,* January 24, 1969.
15. "University Hospital Gets Acne Study Grant," *Philadelphia Bulletin,* July 17, 1970.
16. Fried, "Facing Up to Retin-A®," p. 104.
17. Ibid, p. 150.
18. Lorraine H. Kligman and Albert M. Kligman, "The Effect on Rhino Mouse Skin of Agents which Influence Keratinization and Exfoliation," *Journal of Investigative Dermatology* 73 (1979): 354.
19. Ibid., p. 357.
20. E. G. Thorne, Interoffice Memo Re: Meeting with Dr. Kligman, February 9, 1983. (U.S. Attorney General Office)
21. Interview with George Thorne, January 7, 1997.
22. Sentencing memorandum.

23. E.G. Thorne, Interoffice memo, 1983.
24. James W. Fay, Ortho Interoffice Memo Re: Retin-A® Educational Program, October 29, 1985. (USAGO)
25. Donna T. Pepe, Ortho Pharmaceutical Interoffice Memo, October 7, 1988.
26. Sentencing memorandum of the *United States of America v. Ortho Pharmaceutical Corporation*, March 6, 1995, p. 8. (USAGO)
27. Maripat Sexton, letter to Maria Sisti, assignment editor, WGRZ (NBC), October 8, 1987.
28. James W. Fay, letter to Diane Karsch, April 29, 1986.
29. *MacNeil/Lehrer News Hour*, October 17, 1988, p. 3. (USAGO)
30. Donna T. Pepe, letter to Les Riley, October 26, 1988. (USAGO)
31. Sentencing memorandum, p. 8. (USAGO)
32. Jane Dally, Key Message Points for Media Training, January 12, 1988. (USAGO)
33. Financial response to J. Burke's questions on Retin-A®, February 1, 1988. (USAGO)
34. Sentencing memorandum, p. 10. (USAGO)
35. Sentencing memorandum, p. 10.
36. Leslie N. Vreeland, "The Selling of Retin-A®," *Money* (April 1989): 75.
37. Interview with Diana Zuckerman, November 4, 1996. (USAGO)
38. *University Patents, Inc. v. Albert M. Kligman and Johnson & Johnson*, Civil Action Nos. 89-3525, 90-0422, U. S. District Court for the Eastern District of Pennsylvania, 762 F. Supp. 1212. (USAGO)
39. Ibid., p. 19.
40. Ibid., p. 18.
41. Ibid., p. 18.
42. Ibid., p. 28.
43. Richard Burke, "Penn Suit Puts a New Wrinkle in Retin-A® Case," *Philadelphia Inquirer*, January 23, 1990, p. C1; L. Stuart Ditzen, "As Their Research Brings Results, Universities Discover Patent Problems," *Philadelphia Inquirer*, April 29, 1990, p. G1. (USAGO)
44. Richard Gorelick, "Retin-A® Documents May Shed Light on Government Investigation," *Daily Pennsylvanian*, February 14, 1990.
45. Statement to *60 Minutes,* undated. (USAGO)
46. Sentencing memorandum, p. 15. (USAGO)
47. Ibid., p. 17.
48. Ibid., p. 17.
49. *University Patents, Inc. v. Albert M. Kligman*, p. 27. (USAGO)
50. "Penn Settles Patent Suits on Retin-A®," *Philadelphia Inquirer*, March 6, 1992, p. B6.
51. Jennifer Newman, "Wrinkle Warrior," *American Health* (September 1992): 23.
52. Interview with Alan Lisook, November 9, 1995.
53. Vreeland, "The Selling of Retin-A®," p. 80.
54. Transcript of proceedings, Plea, *United States of America v. Ortho Pharmaceutical Corporation*, U.S. District Court for the District of New Jersey, Criminal No. 95-12, January 11, 1995, p. 15. (USAGO)

55. Transcript of proceedings, Sentencing, *United States of America v. Ortho Pharmaceutical Corporation,* U.S. District Court for the District of New Jersey, Criminal No. 95-12, April 10, 1995, p. 9. (USAGO)
56. Ibid., p. 11.
57. Interview with Kenneth L. Jost, October 31, 1996.
58. *United States of America v. Lester W. Riley, Jr.,* U. S. District Court of New Jersey, Criminal No. 18 USC 371, 1512, and 2, p. 6. (USAGO)
59. Ibid., p. 7.
60. Interview with Faria Mescar, November 27, 1995.
61. Interview with Gerald Wachs, January 7, 1997.
62. Interview with Frederich Urbach.

Chapter Nine

1. Interview with Paul Gross, January 22, 1996.
2. Jay Katz, "The Nuremberg Code and the Nuremberg Trial," *Journal of the American Medical Association* 276, 20 (November 27, 1996): 1662.
3. Ibid., p. 1665.
4. "Citizen Doctor," *Time* (January 13, 1947): 47.
5. "The Green Committee Report," *Journal of the American Medical Association* 136 (1948): 457.
6. David J. Rothman, *Strangers at the Bedside* (New York: Basic Books, 1991), p. 63.
7. *Journal of the American Medical Association* 132 (December 1946): 1090.
8. Henry K. Beecher, "Ethics and Clinical Research," *New England Journal of Medicine* 274, 24 (June 16, 1966): 1360.
9. Interview with Paul R. Gross, January 22, 1996.
10. Interview with A. Bernard Ackerman, September 9, 1996.
11. Jessica Mitford, "Cheaper Than Chimpanzees," *Kind and Usual Punishment* (New York: Alfred A. Knopf, 1973). p. 172.
12. Interview with C. Stuttgen, December 20, 1996.
13. Interview with Frederich Urbach, February 7, 1996.
14. Herman Beerman and Gerald Lazarus, *The Tradition of Excellence: Dermatology at the University of Pennsylvania 1870–1985* (Philadelphia: University of Pennsylvania Press, 1986), pp. 135, 169.
15. Interview with Walter Shelley, January 22, 1996.
16. Ibid.
17. Frederick Weidman, comments on "The Pathogenesis of Tinea Capitis Due to Microsporum Audouini and Microsporum Canis," by Albert M. Kligman, *Journal of Investigative Dermatology* 18, 3 (March 1952): 246.
18. Interview with Paul Gross.
19. Interview with Alex Gougnin. October 2, 1994.
20. Interview with Gerd Plewig, May 22, 1996.
21. Adolph Katz, "Prisoners Volunteer To Save Lives," *Philadelphia Bulletin,* February 27, 1966, p. 1; Burton A. Chardak, "Prisoners Aid Research, 75% Here Act as Medical Guinea Pigs," *Philadelphia Bulletin,* September 18, 1960, p. 5.

22. "The Brutalities of Nazi Physicians," *Journal of the American Medical Association* 132, 12 (November 23, 1946): 714.
23. Interviews with A. Bernard Ackerman.
24. Hans Jonas, "Philosophical Reflections on Experimenting with Human Subjects," in Paul Freund, ed., *Experimentation with Human Subjects* (New York: George Braziller, 1970).

Bibliography

Books

Altman, Lawrence K. Who Goes First? *The Story of Self-Experimentation in Medicine*. New York: Random House, 1987.

Annas, George J., and Grodin, Michael A. *The Nazi Doctors and the Nuremberg Code*. New York: Oxford University Press, 1992.

Basson, Marc D., Rachel E. Lipson, and Doreen L. Ganos, eds. *Troubling Problems in Medical Ethics*. New York: Alan R. Liss, 1981.

Beerman, Herman and Gerald Lazarus. *The Tradition of Excellence: Dermatology at the University of Pennsylvania 1870-1985*. Philadelphia: University of Pennsylvania Press, 1986.

Bennett, James V. *Of Prisoners and Justice*. Washington DC.: U.S. Government Printing Office, 1964.

Caplan, Arthur L., ed. *When Medicine Went Mad*. Totowa, N.J.: Humana Press, 1992.

Childress, James, Gerald Dworkin, Edmund Pellegrino, and Patricia King. *Experimentation with Human Subjects*. Frederick, Md: University Publications of America, 1984.

———. *Informed Consent to Therapy and Experimentation*. Frederick, Md: University Publications of America, 1984.

Ciba Foundation Symposium. *Medical Care of Prisoners and Detainees*. Amsterdam: Associated Scientific Publishers, 1973.

Clegg, Andrew C., III. *An Original Man: The Life and Times of Elijah Muhammad*. New York: St. Martins Press, 1997.

Cole, Leonard A. *Clouds of Secrecy: The Army's Germ Warfare Tests over Populated Areas*. Totowa, N.J.: Rowman and Littlefield, 1988.

———. *The Eleventh Plague*. New York: W. H. Freeman, 1997.

Condon, Richard. *The Manchurian Candidate*. New York: McGraw-Hill, 1959.

Cooter, Roger, ed. *In the Name of the Child: Health Medical Experiments, 1890-1930*. London: Routledge, 1992.

Covert, Norman M. *Cutting Edge: A History of Fort Detrick, Maryland, 1943-1993*. Fort Detrick: Public Affairs Office, 1993.

Cressey, Donald R., ed. *The Prison.* New York: Holt, Rinehart and Winston, 1961.

DiIulio, John J., Jr. *No Escape.* New York: Basic Books, 1991.

Etheridge, Elizabeth W. *The Butterfly Caste.* Westport, CT: Greenwood Publishing, 1972.

Evans, Donald, and Martyn Evans. *A Decent Proposal: Ethical Review of Clinical Research.* New York: Wiley, 1996.

Faden, Ruth R., and Tom L. Beauchamp. *A History and Theory of Informed Consent.* New York: Oxford University Press, 1986.

Faden, Ruth R. et al., eds. *Final Report—Advisory Committee on Human Radiation Experiments.* Pittsburgh: U.S. Government Printing Office, 1995.

Fox, Renee C. *Experiment Perilous.* Glencoe, Ill.: The Free Press, 1959.

Freund, Paul A., ed. *Experimentation with Human Beings.* New York: George Braziller, 1970.

Friedman, Lawrence M. *Crime and Punishment in America.* New York: Basic Books, 1993.

Gotz, Aly, Peter Chroust, and Christian Pross. *Cleansing the Fatherland.* Baltimore: Johns Hopkins Press, 1994.

Goulden, Paula, and Benjamin Naitove. *Medical Science and the Law.* New York: Facts on File Publishers, 1984.

Gray, Bradford H. *Human Subjects in Medical Experimentation.* New York: Wiley & Sons, 1975.

Grodin, Michael A., and Leonard H. Glantz, eds. *Children as Research Subjects.* New York: Oxford University Press, 1994.

Harris, Sheldon H. *Factories of Death.* New York: Routledge, 1994.

Harvey, A. McGehee. *Science at the Bedside: Clinical Research in American Medicine 1905–1945.* Baltimore: Johns Hopkins University, 1981.

Jacobs, James B. *Stateville.* Chicago: University of Chicago Press, 1977.

Jones, James H. *Bad Blood.* New York: The Free Press, 1993.

Katz, Jay. *Experimentation with Human Beings.* New York: Russell Sage Foundation, 1972.

Keve, Paul W. *A History of U.S. Federal Corrections.* Carbondale: Southern Illinois University Press, 1991.

Kraut, Alan M. *Silent Travelers: Germs, Genes, and the "Immigrant Menace."* New York: Basic Books, 1994.

Lederer, Susan. *Subjected to Science.* Baltimore: Johns Hopkins University Press, 1995.

———. "Orphans as Guinea Pigs: American Children and Medical Experimenters, 1890-1930." In Roger Cooter, In *The Name of the Child:*

Health and Welfare, 1880–1940. New York: Routledge, 1992.

Leopold, Nathan F., Jr. *Life Plus 99 Years.* Garden City, N.Y.: Doubleday, 1958.

Levine, Robert J. *Ethics and Regulation of Clinical Research.* Baltimore: Urban and Schwartzenberg, 1981.

Lifton, Robert Jay. *The Nazi Doctors.* New York: Basic Books, 1986.

Maibach, Howard I., ed. *Occupational and Industrial Dermatology.* Chicago: Yearbook Medical Publishers, 1987.

Marks, John. *The Search for the Manchurian Candidate.* New York: Norton, 1979.

McNeill, Paul M. *The Ethics and Politics of Human Experimentation.* Hong Kong: Cambridge University Press, 1993.

Meyer, Peter B. *Drug Experiments on Prisoners.* Lexington, Mass.: Lexington Books, 1976.

Mitford, Jessica. *Kind and Usual Punishment.* New York: Knopf, 1973.

Moore, Thomas J. *Deadly Medicine.* New York: Simon & Schuster, 1995.

Pappworth, M. H. *Human Guinea Pigs.* Boston: Beacon Press, 1967.

Pillsbury, Donald M., Walter B. Shelley, and Albert M. Kligman. *Dermatology.* Philadelphia: W. B. Saunders, 1956.

Proctor, Robert N. *Racial Hygiene: Medicine Under the Nazis.* Cambridge, Mass.: Harvard University Press, 1988.

Prout, Curtis, and Robert Ross. *Care and Punishment.* Pittsburgh: University of Pittsburgh Press, 1988.

Reiser, Stanley Joel, Arthur J. Dyck, and William J. Curran. *Ethics in Medicine.* Cambridge: MIT Press, 1977.

Rothman, David J. *Strangers at the Bedside.* New York: Basic Books, 1991.

Rothman, David J., and Sheila M. Rothman. *The Willowbrook Wars.* New York: Harper & Row, 1984.

Silverman, William A. *Human Experimentation.* New York: Oxford University Press, 1985.

Squire, Amos O. *Sing Sing Doctor.* New York: Garden City Publishing, 1937.

Szymansky, Frederic J. *Centenial History of American Dermatological Association.* Philadelphia: W. B. Saunders, 1956.

Thomas, Evan. *The Very Best Men.* New York: Simon & Schuster, 1996.

Turner, Patricia A. *I Heard It Through The Grapevine.* Berkeley: University of California Press, 1993.

Vallenstein, Elliot S. *Great and Desperate Cures.* New York: Basic Books, 1986.

Weisse, Allen B. *Medical Odysseys.* New Brunswick, N.J.: Rutgers University Press, 1991.

Williams, Peter, and David Wallace. Unit 731: *The Japanese Army's Secret of Secrets.* London: Hodder and Stoughton, 1989.

GOVERNMENT DOCUMENTS

The following documents were obtained through extensive use of the Freedom of Information Act:

Central Intelligence Agency: Files concerning Projects MKULTRA and OFTEN on the agency's long-standing interest and involvement with mind-control experiments.

Department of the Army: Files of the U.S. Army's Medical Research Laboratories located at Edgewood Arsenal on the use of prisoners as research subjects for chemical warfare experiments.

Environmental Protection Agency: Files related to the agency's investigation of dioxin experiments at Holmesburg Prison in Philadelphia.

Food and Drug Administration: Files related to the investigation and sanction of Dr. Albert M. Kligman and his studies on dimethyl-sulfoxide at Holmesburg Prison in 1966.

Nuclear Regulatory Commission: Files of the Atomic Energy Commission related to the application and use of radioactive materials at Holmesburg Prison in the 1960s.

JOURNAL ARTICLES

Anderson, J.A.D., and I. H. Stokoe. "Vitamin A in Acne Vulgaris." *British Medical Journal* (August 3, 1963).

Arnold, John D., Daniel C. Martin, and Sarah E. Boyer. "A Study of One Prison Population and its Responses to Medical Research." *Annals of the New York Academy of Sciences* 169 (January 21, 1970).

"Baldness Breakthrough." Editorial. *Journal of the American Medical Association* 191, 7 (February 15, 1965).

Beecher, Henry K. "Ethics and Clinical Research." *New England Journal of Medicine* 274, 24 (June 16, 1966).

Berg, Jessica W. "Legal and Ethical Complexities of Consent with Cognitively Impaired Research Subjects: Proposed Guidelines." *The Journal of Law, Medicine, and Ethics* 24, 1 (Spring 1994).

Besley, S. H. "Heart at Death." *Life* (November 7, 1938).

"Biomedical Ethics and the Shadow of Nazism." *Hastings Center Report* (August 1976).

Bleiberg, Jacob, Marven Wallen, Rodger Brodkin, and Irving Applebaum. "Industrial Acquired Porphyria." *Archives of Dermatology* 89 (1964).

Brandt, Allan M., and Lara Freidenfelds. "Research Ethics after World War II: The Insular Culture of Biomedicine." *Kennedy Institute of Ethics Journal* 6, 3

(September 1996).

Buchanan, Allen. "The Controversy over Retrospective Moral Judgements." *Kennedy Institute of Ethics Journal* 6, 3 (1996).

Caplan, Arthur L. "When Evil Intrudes." *Hastings Center Report* (November 1992).

Cherin, Eli. "Richard Pearson Strong and the Iatrogenic Plague Disaster in Bilibid Prison, Manila, 1906." *Reviews of Infectious Diseases* 11, 6 (November 1989).

Coombs, Francis P., and Thomas Butterworth. "Atypical Keratosis Pilaris." *Archives of Dermatology and Syphilology* 62, 2 (August 1950).

Edgar, Harold, and David J. Rothman. "The Institutional Review Board and Beyond: Future Challenges to the Ethics of Human Experimentation." *Milbank Quarterly* 73, 4 (1995).

Epstein, W. L. and A. M. Kligman. "The Pathogenesis of Milia and Benign Tumors of the Skin." *Journal of Investigative Dermatology* 56 (1956).

———. and A. M. Kligman. "Pathogenesis of Eosinophilia Pneumonitis." *Journal of the American Medical Association* 152 (1956).

———, and A. M. Kligman. "Epithelial Cysts in Buried Human Skin." *Archives of Dermatology* 76 (1957).

Fulton, James E., Jr., Paul Gross, Chalmers E. Cornelius, and Albert M. Kligman. "Darier's Disease." *Archives of Dermatology* 98 (October 1968).

Fulton, James E., Jr., Gerd Plewig, and Albert M. Kligman. "Effect of Chocolate on Acne Vulgaris." *Journal of the American Medical Association* 210, 11 (December 15, 1969).

Goldschmidt, Herbert, and Albert M. Kligman. "Experimental Inoculation of Humans with Ectodermotropic Viruses." *Journal of Investigative Dermatology* 31, 3 (September 1958).

Heller, Melvin. "Problems and Prospects in the Use of Prison Inmates for Medical Experimentation." *Prison Journal* 57, 1 (Spring 1967).

Hodges, Robert E., and William B. Bean. "The Uses of Prisoners for Medical Research." *Journal of the American Medical Association* 202, 6 (November 6, 1967.)

Katz, Jay. "The Nuremberg Code and the Nuremberg Trial." *Journal of the American Medical Association* 276, 20 (November 27, 1996).

Kemp, Thomas S., and Albert M. Kligman. "The Effect of X-Rays on Experimentally Produced Acute Contact Dermatitis." *Journal of Investigative Dermatitis* 23 (1954).

Kevorkian, Jack. "A Brief History of Experimentation on Condemned and Executed Humans." *Journal of the National Medical Association* 77, 3 (1985).

Kligman, Albert M. "Application of Potassium Hydroxide to the Skin as an Aid in Direct Examination of Scales for Fungi." *Archives of Dermatology & Syphilology* 63 (February 1951).

———. "The Pathogenesis of Tinea Capitis Due to Microsporum Audouini and Microsporum Canis." *Journal of Investigative Dermatology* 18, 3, (March 1952).

———. "Plastic Band-Aids for Patch Testing." *Archives of Dermatology* 75 (May 1957).

———. "Poison Ivy (Rhus) Dermatitis." *Archives of Dermatology* 77 (February 1958).

———. "Pathologic Dynamics of Human Hair Loss." *Archives of Dermatology* 83 (February 1961).

———. "Topical Pharmacology and Toxicology of Dimethyl Sulfoxide." Part I. *Journal of the American Medical Association* 193, 10 (September 6, 1965).

———. "Dimethyl Sulfoxide-A Correction." *Journal of the American Medical Association* 197, 13 (September 26, 1966).

Kligman, Albert M., and W. Ward Anderson. "Evaluation of Current Methods for the Local Treatment of Tinea Capitis." *Journal of Investigative Dermatology* 16 (March 1961).

Kligman, Albert M., and Reinhard Breit. "The Identification of Phototoxic Drugs by Human Assay." *Journal of Investigative Dermatology* 51, 2 (1968).

Kligman, Albert M., and Edward D. DeLamater. "The Immunology of the Human Mycoses." *Annual Review of Microbiology* 4 (1950).

Kligman, Albert M. and W. L. Epstein. "Suppression of Local Allergic Reaction with Hydrocortisone." *Journal of Allergy* 27 (1956).

———. "Warts Treated with Cantharidin." *Archives of Dermatology* 77 (1958).

Kligman, Albert M., and Dorothy Ginsberg. "Immunity of the Adult Scalp to Infection with Microsporum Audouini." *Journal of Investigative Dermatology* 14 (May 1950).

Kligman, Albert M., and I. Willis. "A New Formula for Depigmenting Human Skin." *Archives of Dermatology* (1975).

Kligman, Albert M., and W. M. Wooding. "A Method for the Measurement and Evaluation of Irritants on Human Skin." *Journal of Investigative Dermatology* 49, 1 (1967).

Kligman, Albert M., James E. Fulton, Jr., and Gerd Plewig. "Topical Vitamin A Acid in Acne Vulgaris." *Archives of Dermatology* 99 (April 1969).

Kligman, Albert M., H. Mescon, and E. D. DeLamater. "The Hotchkiss-McManus Stain for the Histopathic Diagnosis of Fungus Disease." *American Journal of Clinical Pathology* (January 1951).

Kligman, Albert M., Otto Mills, James J. Leyden, Paul Gross, Herbert B. Allen, and Robert I. Rudolph. "Oral Vitamin A in Acne Vulgaris." *International Journal of Dermatology* (May 1981).

Kligman, Albert M., D. M. Pillsbury, and H. Mescon. "Improved Technique for Diagnosing Ringworm Infections and Moniliasis." *Journal of the American Medical Association* (August 25, 1951).

Kligman, Albert M., Gerd Plewig, and Otto Mills, Jr. "Topically Applied Tretinoin for Senile Comedones." *Archives of Dermatology* 104 (October 1971).

Kligman, Lorraine H., and Albert M. Kligman. "The Effect on Rhino Mouse Skin of Agents which Influence Keratinization and Exfoliation." *Journal of Investigative Dermatology* 73 (1979).

Maguire, H. C., and A. M. Kligman. "Norwegian Scabies." *Archives of Dermatology* 82 (1960).

———. "Histopathology of Common Male Baldness." Proceedings of the twelfth Congress of Dermatology, 1963.

Maibach, Howard I., and Albert M. Kligman. "The Biology of Experimental Human Cutaneous Moniliasis." *Archives of Dermatology* 85 (1962).

Martin, Daniel C., John D. Arnold, T. F. Zimmerman, and Robert Rickart. "Human Subjects in Clinical Research—A Report of Three Studies." *New England Journal of Medicine* 279, 26 (December 26, 1968).

Mastroianni, Anna, and Jeffrey Kann. "Remedies for Human Subjects of Cold War Research: Recommendations of Advisory Committee." *Journal of Law, Medicine, and Ethics.* 24,2 (Summer 1996).

McDonald, John C. "Why Prisoners Volunteer to be Experimental Subjects." *Journal of the American Medical Association* 202, 6 (1967).

Moreno, Jonathan D., and Susan E. Lederer. "Revising the History of Cold War Research Ethics." *Kennedy Institute of Ethics Journal* 6, 3 (September 1996).

O'Hara, John L. "The Most Unforgettable Character I've Met." *Reader's Digest* (May 1948).

Papa, Christopher, and Albert M. Kligman. "Stimulation of Hair Growth by Topical Application of Androgens." *Journal of the American Medical Association* 191, 7 (February 15, 1965).

———, and Albert M. Kligman. "The Behavior of Melanocytes in Inflamation." *Journal of Investigative Dermatology* 45, 6 (1965).

Papa, Christopher M., D. M. Carter, and A. M. Kligman. "The Effect of Autotransplantation on the Progression or Reversibility of Aging in Human Skin." *Journal of Investigative Dermatology* 54, 3 (1970).

Pappworth, M. H. "Human Guinea Pigs." *British Medical Journal* 301 (1990).

Pawson, Beverly A. "History of Retinoids." *Journal of the American Academy of Dermatology* 6, 4 (April 1982).

Poland, Alan P., Donald Smith, Gerald Metter, and Paul Possick. "A Health Survey of Workers in a 2, 4D and 2,4,5-T Plant." *Archives of Environmental Health* 22 (March 1971).

Rebora, Alfredo, Richard R. Marples, and Albert M. Kligman. "Experimental Infection with Candida Albicans." *Archives of Dermatology* 108 (July 1973).

Rothman, David J. "Henry Beecher Revisited." *The New England Journal of Medicine* 317, 19 (November 7, 1987).

Rubin, Jeffrey S. "Breaking Into the Prison: Conducting a Medical Research Project." *American Journal of Psychiatry* 133, 2 (February 1976).

Scully, John P., and Albert M. Kligman. "Coincident Infection of a Human and Anthropoid with Microsporum Audouini." *Archives of Dermatology and Syphilology* (October 1951).

Shehadeh, N. H., and Albert M. Kligman. "The Bacteriology of Acne." *Archives of Dermatology* 88, 6 (1963).

Shelley, Walter B., and Albert M. Kligman. "The Experimental Production of Acne by Penta and Herachlorcnaphthalenes." *Archives of Dermatology* 75 (May 1957).

Shellow, William V. R., and Albert M. Kligman. "An Attempt to Produce Elastosis in Aged Human Skin by Means of Ultraviolet Irradiation." *Journal of Investigative Dermatology* 50, 3 (1968).

Shubin, Seymour. "Research Behind Bars." *The Sciences* (January 1981).

Singh, Gurmohan, Richard R. Marples, and Albert M. Kligman. "Experimental Staphylococcus Aureus Infection in Humans." *Journal of Investigative Dermatology* 57, 3 (1971).

Stanley, L. L. "Testicular Substance Implantation." *Endocrinology* 5 (1921).

———. "An Analysis of One Thousand Testicular Substance Implantations." *Endocrinology* 6 (1922).

Straumfjord, Jonathan V. "Vitamin A: Its Effects on Acne." *Northwest Medicine* 42 (August 1943).

Strauss, John S., and Albert M. Kligman. "Experimental Study of Tinea Pedis and Onychomycosis of the Foot." *Archives of Dermatology* 76 (1957).

———. "Distribution of Skin Doses Over Scalp in Therapy of Tinea Capitis with Superficial X-Rays." *Archives of Dermatology & Syphilology* 70 (July 1954).

Strauss, John S., and Albert M. Kligman. "Acne: Observations on Dermabrasion and the Anatomy of the Acne Pit." *Archives of Dermatology & Syphilology* 74 (1956).

Strauss, John S., and Albert M. Kligman. "The Pathologic Dynamics of Acne Vulgaris." *Archives of Dermatology* 82 (1960).

Weidman, Fred D., and Frederic A. Glass. "Dermatophytosis and other Forms of Intertriginous Dermatitis of the Feet." *Archives of Dermatology and Syphilology* 52, 3, (March 1946).

Weyers, Wolfgang. "Dermatology and Dermatopathology Under the Swastika." *Dermatopathology* I, 4 (October/December 1995).

Wharton, Don. "Prisoners Who Volunteer Blood, Flesh, and Their Lives." *American Mercury* 79 (1954).

Willis, Isaac, and Albert M. Kligman. "Photocontact Allergic Reactions." *Archives of Dermatology* 100 (November 1969).

MAGAZINE ARTICLES

Adams, Aileen, and Geoffrey Cowan. "The Human Guinea Pig: How We Test New Drugs." *World* (December 5, 1972).

Brown, Chip. "The Science Club Serves its Country." *Esquire* (December 1994).

"Cancer by the Needle." *Newsweek* (June 4, 1956).

"Cancer Volunteers." *Time* (February 25, 1957).

"Citizen Doctor." *Time* (January 13, 1947).

"Drug Tests Behind Bars." *Business Week* (June 27, 1964).

Fleeson, Lucinda. "Saving Face." *Philadelphia Inquirer Magazine* (April 10, 1988).

Fried, Stephen. "Facing Up to Retin-A." *Philadelphia Magazine* (April 1996).

"Investigating the Investigator." *Time.* (August 1966).

Mitford, Jessica. "Experiments Behind Bars." *Atlantic Monthly* (January 1973).

Newman, Jennifer. "Wrinkle Warrior." *American Health* (September 1992).

O'Donnell, Paul. "Fallout of an Invisible War." *Newsweek* (July 25, 1994).

"Poison Ivy Picker of Pennypack Park." *Life* (September 5, 1955).

"Volunteers Behind Bars." *Time* (July 12, 1963).

Vreeland, Leslie N. "The Selling of Retin-A." *Money* (April 1989).

LEGAL CASES

Robert Crew, Leodus Jones, George Askew, and Earl Harris v. The Dow Chemical Company et al., United States District Court, Eastern District of Pennsylvania, No. 81-4824.

Roach v. Kligman, Civil Action No. 73-2428, April 30, 1976.

William Smith v. Albert Kligman, Ivy Research, Solomon McBride, Trustees of the University of Pennyslvania, Dow Chemical, Philadelphia Prisons and the City of Philadelphia, Court of Common Pleas, Philadelphia, January 1983.

James Walker and Shirley Walker v. Albert Kligman, Ivy Research Laboratories,

Trustees of the University of Pennsylvania and the City of Philadelphia, Court of Common Pleas, Philadelphia, September 1979.

University Patents, Inc. v. Albert M. Kligman and Johnson & Johnson, Civil Action Nos. 89-3525, 90-0422, United States District Court for the Eastern District of Pennsylvania, 762 F. Supp. 1212.

United States of America v. Lester W. Riley, Jr., United States District Court of New Jersey, Criminal No. 18 USC 371, 1512, and 2, p. 6.

United States of America v. Ortho Pharmaceutical Corporation, United States District Court for the District of New Jersey, Criminal No. 95-12, January 11, 1995, p. 17.

United States of America v. Karl Brandt et al. Trials of War Criminals before the Nuremberg Military Tribunals under Control Council Law, No. 10, June 13, 1947, A-MJ-23-2 Gross (Brown) Court I, p. 9171.

INTERVIEWS

Prisoners

Ahad, Simon Khaadim. Interview with author at S. C. I. Graterford, April 28, 1994.

Allison, Willie (pseudonym). Interview with the author at S. C. I. Graterford, April 28, 1994.

Biose, Jay (pseudonym). Interview with the author, October 1995.

Bradley, George. Interview with the author at S. C. I. Graterford, April 28, 1994.

Butler, Al (pseudonym). Interview with author at S. C. I. Graterford, May 26, 1994.

Crawford, Raymond. Interview with author at S. C. I. Graterford, April 28, 1994.

Epps, Mathew. Interview with author at S. C. I. Graterford, April 28,1994.

Hollick, Andy (pseudonym). Interview with author, May 18, 1994.

Jones, Leodus. Interview with author, May 18, 1994.

Keenan, Ron (pseudonym). Interview with author at S. C. I. Graterford, October 21, 1994.

Lawson, Allan. Interview with author, June 14, 1994.

Lewis, James. Interview with author at S. C. I. Graterford, July 7, 1994.

Lincoln, Steve (pseudonym). Letter to author from S. C. I. Graterford, April 11, 1994.

Lopinson, Jack. Interview with author at S. C. I. Graterford, March 14, 1994.

Mancini, Rick (pseudonym). Interview with author at S. C. I. Graterford, April 28, 1994.

McCafferty, William. Interview with author at S. C. I. Graterford, April 28, 1994.

McGevren, Tom (pseudonym). Interview with author, September 26, 1994.

O'Maley, Bubba (pseudonym) Sr. Letter to author from Delaware Correctional

Center, October 18, 1994.

Ponton, Withers. Interview with author at S. C. I. Graterford, April 28, 1994.

Porter, George (pseudonym). Telephone interview with author from S. C. I. Graterford, June 1, 1994.

Robb, William (pseudonym). Letter to author from S. C. I. Pittsburgh, undated.

Sellner, Darren (pseudonym). Interview with author, September 20, 1994.

Sims, Thomas. Interview with author, May 3, 1994.

Walker, Ralph (pseudonym). Telephone interview from S. C. I.Graterford, June 1, 1994.

Williams, Johnnie (pseudonym). Interviews with author, beginning May 19, 1994.

Zabala, Al. Interviews with author at S. C. I. Graterford, March 16, 1994, and on furlough April 27, 1994.

Correctional Personnel

Brame, Hank. Telephone interview with author, March 3, 1994.

Dade, Joseph. Interview with author, April 27, 1994.

Foxworth, Fred. Telephone interview with author, June 7, 1994.

Goodman, Fred. Telephone interview with author, June 1994.

Gomez, Ron. Interview with author, June 1994.

Gougnin, Alex. Interview with author, October 2, 1994.

Hightower, Willie. Telephone interview with author, June 2, 1994.

Kinslow, James. Interview with author at Holmesburg Prison, March 31, 1994.

Lyons, Edmund. Interview with author, April 6, 1994.

Miller, Curtis. Telephone interview with author, June, 1994.

Williams, Leroy. Interview with the author, May 6, 1997.

Physicians

Ackerman, A. Bernard. Interviews with author, February 1, 1996-July 25, 1997.

Baer, Rudolph. Telephone interview with author, February 5, 1996.

Boxer, Arthur. Interview with author at S. C. I. Graterford, July 20, 1994.

Calesnick, Benjamin. Interviews with author, beginning November 27, 1995.

Cahn, Burt. Telephone interview with author, February 8, 1996.

Cahn, Milton. Interview with author, February 8, 1996.

Corcoran, Joseph. Telephone interview with author, January 3, 1997.

Cornelius, Chalmers. Telephone interview with author, November 25, 1996.

Epstein, William. Telephone interview with author, July 25, 1995.

Franzblau, Michael. Interview with author, December 10, 1996.

Frost, Phillip. Telephone interview with author, February 26, 1996.

Gross, Paul. Interview with the author, January 22, 1996.

Guy, Edward. Interview with author at Philadelphia Detention Center, October 1994.

Heller, Melvin. Interview with author, September 20, 1994.

Kelsey, Francis. Telephone interview with author, January 12, 1995.

Ketchum, James. Telephone interviews with author, beginning February 15, 1995.

Kligman, Albert M. Telephone interview with author, January 10, 1995.

Lisook, Alan B. Telephone interview with author, January 13, 1995.

Livingood, Clarence. Telephone interview with author, March 20, 1996.

Maguire, Henry C. Telephone interview with author.

Maibach, Howard I. Telephone interview with author, July 25, 1995.

Mescar, Faria. Interview with author, November 27, 1995.

Parrish, Lawrence C. Interviews with author, beginning December 18, 1996.

Plewig, Gerd. Telephone interview with author, May 22, 1996.

Rawnsley Howard M. Telephone interview with author, September 27, 1994.

Shelley, Walter. Telephone interview with author, January 22, 1996.

Sidell, Frederick. Telephone interview with author, December 15, 1994.

Southam, Chester M. Interview with author, October 3, 1996.

Start, Aron. Telephone interview with author, May, 1994.

Stuttgen, C. Telephone interview with author, December 20, 1996.

Thorne, George. Telephone interview with author, January 1, 1997.

Troyan, Beatrice. Interview with author, November 14, 1996.

Van Scott, Eugene. Telephone interview with author, February 7, 1996.

Wachs, Gerald. Telephone interview with author, January 7, 1997.

Weitzman, Sigmund. Telephone interview with author, May 10, 1994.

Wilson, John F. Telephone interview with author, March 3, 1997.

Willis, Isaac. Telephone interview with author, February 2, 1996.

Witkowski, Joseph. Telephone interview with author, January 3, 1997.

Wood, Margaret Grey. Telephone interview with author, February 17, 1997.

ADDITIONAL INTERVIEWS

Anderson, Brian. Telephone interview with author, November 1995.

Annas, George. Telephone interview with author, May 17, 1996.

Antosh, Lou. Telephone interview with author, October 3, 1994.

Arter, Karen. Telephone interview with author, September 18, 1996.

Bechelheimer, Robert. Telephone interview with author, February 2, 1996.

Becroft, Pricilla. Telephone interview with author, November 24, 1994.

Blackwell, Lucien. Interview with author, October 24, 1996.

Bowen, Angela. Telephone interview with author, December 30, 1996.

Bronstein, Alvin. Telephone interview with author, June 22, 1995.

Byrne, Lawrence. Interview with author, December 7, 1994.

Caplan, Aethur Interview with Author, March 30, 1994.

Capron, Alexander. Telephone interview with author, September 30, 1994.

Carpenter, Victor H. Telephone interview with author, September 1994.

Carter, Peggy. Telephone interview with author, January 28, 1996.

Chalfin, Paul. Telephone interview with author, October 12, 1994.

Cox, Spencer. Telephone interview with author, June 19, 1997.

Davido, Frank. Telephone interview with author, February 20, 1996.

Fox, Renee. Telephone interview with author, September 19, 1996.

Goldberg, Paul. Telephone interview with author, November 13, 1995.

Greenfield, Steven. Telephone interview with author, December 22, 1994.

Hepp, Jack, Jr. Telephone interview with author, May 12, 1996.

Humphrey, Mattie. Telephone interview with author, February 4, 1997.

Johnson, Seymour M., Jr. Telephone interview with author, September 1994.

Johnston, Norman. Interview with author, November 6, 1996.

Jost, Kenneth L. Telephone interview with author, October 31, 1996.

Kasten, Frederich H. Telephone interview with author, May 13, 1996.

Katz, Alan. Telephone interview with author, October 7, 1994.

Kneebone, Leon. Telephone interview with author, January 22, 1996.

Koren, Edward. Telephone interview with author, June 1995.

Lebowitz, Harriet. Telephone interview with author, November 12, 1996.

Levitt, Albert. Telephone interview with author, September 12, 1994.

Loev, Bernard. Telephone interview with author, August 12, 1996.

Maeder, Thomas. Telephone interview with author, January 18, 1995.

McBride, Solomon. Telephone interview with author, December 8, 1994.

McCluney, Robert. Telephone interview with author, May 21, 1994.

Mills, Otto. Telephone interview with author, February 5, 1996.

Mirarchi, Charles. Interview with author, June 28, 1994.

Mishkin, Barbara. Telephone interview with author, November 12, 1996.

Mitford, Jessica. Telephone interview with author, October 23, 1995.

Mueller, Gerhard. Telephone interview with author, October 11, 1994.

Packman, Elias, Interview with author, March 19, 1996.

Ray, Artis. Telephone interview with the author, September 1994.

Raymon, Jean. Telephone interview with author, January 19, 1996.

Robbins, Jack. Telephone interview with author, January 6, 1997.

Rowe, Verald Kieth. Telephone interview with author, April 17, 1994.

Rubolina, James. Interview with author, March 1995.

Rudovsky, David. Interview with author, May 13, 1994.

Samitz, Doris. Telephone interview with author, June 27, 1995.

Schwartz, Lindsey. Telephone interview with author, May 1997.

Scott, Sheila. Telephone interview with author, January 10, 1995.

Shouler, Tom. Interview with author, June 14, 1997.

Sielaff, Allyn. Telephone interview with author, December 7, 1994.

Smith, Cecil O., Jr. Telephone interview with author, September 22, 1994.

Triol, Calvin. Interview with author, October 10, 1994.

Willson, Scott. Interview with the author, December 1994.

Wolfgang, Marvin. Telephone interview with author, September 1994.

Zillmer, Erich. Interview with author, March 27, 1996.

Zuckerman, Diana. Telephone interview with author, November 4, 1996.

Index